HOMEOPATHY
FOR TODAY

HOMEOPATHY
FOR TODAY

Family Friendly, Simple & Safe Healing

David Robert Card

Kalindi Press
Chino Valley, Arizona

Cover Design: Hohm Press

Interior Design and Layout: Becky Fulker, Kubera Book Design, Prescott, Arizona

Library of Congress Control Number: 2023930423

ISBN: 978-1-935826-60-6
E-book: 978-1-935826-61-3

Kalindi Press
P.O. Box 4410
Chino Valley, AZ 86323
800-381-2700
http://www.kalindipress.com

This book was printed in the U.S.A. on recycled, acid-free paper using soy ink.

To my wonderful wife Teresa, and my faithful clients

Acknowledgements

Many thanks to the myriad of clients I have consulted with over these last many years, and the great successes we have experienced using homeopathy. My gratitude to Robin Murphy, N.D. for my training and his great insights. Thanks to all my family, especially my wife Teresa, for their continued support. I'm also grateful for the support of my homeopathic study group and all their questions and discussions as we studied together. Thanks and gratitude to Linda Fulton, for organizing all my thoughts and intents into this work.

Contents

Chapter 3: MATERIA MEDICA: REMEDY GUIDE WITH KEYNOTES AND SYMPTOMS

Foreword

I first became interested in homeopathy when, as a young mother, my son had infections and medical issues that modern medicine wasn't able to fix. Learning that there were other modalities that were not only safer, but could help him heal quicker, and without as many complications, I began my study of homeopathy and herbal treatments that would span decades. Over these years, I have seen countless family, friends, and clients find relief to their physical and emotional ailments through the modalities taught in this book. Being able to study under and work with Dave the past few years, I have seen that he has a fundamental grasp on homeopathy as a whole, that can bless the lives of everyone who comes into contact with his teachings, whether you are a beginner or highly advanced in your studies. Because of this book's simplicity, readers will have an opportunity to adopt these principles into their own lives to restore health quickly and easily to themselves and their loved ones.

—Heidi L. Parker, BCTN (Board Certified Traditional Naturopath)

Introduction

In my practice as a homeopath, I consult with people who want to take care of their family's health and be as self-sufficient as possible. I wrote this book for individuals and parents who want to treat common health issues in their families, using homeopathic remedies. Most people don't have access to a homeopath at a moment's notice, when health issues arise. This book will give you access to information needed to help you or your family members use homeopathic remedies right now. Anyone can benefit from homeopathy regardless of their age, gender, condition of pregnancy, or if using medications.

Along with my greater than forty years of experience in personal use and consulting with thousands of clients, the information in this book has also been gleaned from over two-hundred years of human homeopathic provings and documented "cured" cases. Homeopathic medicines have been proven to work in more than 2,000 double-blind scientific studies around the world. These successes will benefit you and your family. To make it easy for you, I will not be using excessive medical terminology or jargon, so you will be able to understand how to use homeopathy, quick and simple.

If you are one who seeks safe, inexpensive, effective healing without the side effects of medications, or drug interactions, you are in the right place. This book is centered on the time-honored remedies that most people can have on hand or can obtain easily at a low cost. These chosen homeopathic remedies have been proven, in my practice, to give rapid results.

What are the benefits of using homeopathic remedies? To begin with, they are safe for everyone; you can take them even if you are taking other medicines, such as over-the-counter or prescription medications; they taste good, an added bonus when giving to children; you can obtain them easily through your local health-food store, or online with reputable companies; they are inexpensive! But, the greatest benefit comes when you take the remedy that matches most closely to your symptoms, and your symptoms just go away, either rapidly or gradually. (We call it the *simillimum*, or the most similar. See Homeopathic Principle 1 in Chapter 1).

Using homeopathy is as simple as matching the symptoms of the person with the right homeopathic remedy, is as close an agreement as possible, which will make a profound difference. To see the amazing results in thousands of my clients over the years has been truly gratifying. In my homeopathic practice, many times a client would return a few weeks after our consultation and tell me how other symptoms or health issues had cleared up, besides the one we were working on. Homeopathic medicine can deal with healing underlying health issues. It's true! These remedies sometimes defy the beliefs of Western medicine in how the body heals. Where Western medicine has no answers for some people, there are many health issues for which homeopathy works. We don't always know the mechanisms, but we see the results!

To benefit most from this book, learn the simple truths of homeopathy in the first chapter: Homeopathy: What It Is and How to Use It.

Next, in the Conditions Repertory chapter you will find common health conditions with brief descriptions of the symptoms of each condition, including reasonable outcomes for most people. Since many clients ask, I offer some reasonable estimates of the timeframe for recognizable results. I have heard thousands of success stories from my clients over the years, and have included a few of them here so you will have the courage to try homeopathic remedies yourself, and write your own success stories.

In the Materia Medica or Remedy Guide chapter, I give a detailed list of the most common symptoms (head to toe) that each remedy addresses. These include Keynotes, which are specific symptoms—usually three or so—that are the most common for that remedy and will direct you to the matching remedy quickly and accurately. To find the right remedy even faster, look to the Quick Reference chapter that has guides to Keynotes (leading symptoms), top remedies, and more.

HOW TO USE THIS BOOK

- **Learn about Homeopathy and How to Use It**
  In Chapter 1 you will learn how homeopathy came about, and how to use and care for your homeopathic remedies.

- **Find the Right Remedy** (Simillimum or like-cures-like)
  Look in Chapter 2 to find a condition or symptoms you are experiencing—the one or ones that are most important to you right now. Remember, injuries should always be treated first. In each condition you will find several remedies indicated for that condition, with descriptions of leading symptoms. Choose the remedy that most closely matches the symptoms you are experiencing. If there is more than one remedy that fits your situation, that's okay. (See: Using or Making Homeopathic Combinations in Chapter 1.)

- **Verify the Right Remedy in the Materia Medica (Remedy Guide)**
  Chapter 3 will give you more details on the homeopathic remedy that matches your symptoms the most, including: keynotes—the guiding symptoms for that remedy; physical and mental/emotional symptoms; modalities (when your symptoms are better or worse, such as the time of day, temperature changes, etc.), and more. Remember, if there is more than one remedy that fits, it is just fine to take more than one remedy at a time.

- **Use the Quick-Reference** chapter if you are pressed for time. Check out these guides that can quickly lead you to the remedy most similar to your needs with a symptom, keynote, modality, or top remedy.

- **Before Moving Forward, Never Stop Your Prescription Medications.** As conditions improve, get with your healthcare provider to reduce medications.

- **Take the Remedy.** Take the single remedy or combination that best fits your condition or symptoms. Homeopathic remedies should be taken 5-10 minutes before or after eating or drinking. Use potencies of 6C – 30C, two to three times a day. If it is an injury or emergency, you can use a 200C potency, and call for help (emergency personnel) if needed.

- **Look for Improvement.** If it is a recent condition (acute), expect to see gradual or quick results within hours to a few days. If it is a longstanding (chronic) condition, it can improve gradually in days, weeks, or months. Be patient. If not seeing improvement, try another remedy or make a combination of remedies (see Chapter 1 for more information).

- **See Your Healthcare Provider** if your symptoms get worse or you are not feeling well.

- **See a Homeopath** if your condition doesn't improve, so they can "take your case" and find a true simillimum for you.

NOTES TO THE READER:

- The remedies found in this book are the most commonly used, especially in my homeopathic practice. They should be readily available in health food stores or online (always use reputable sources). This book is not a comprehensive work in homeopathy as there's a vast amount of information written elsewhere. My goal in this book is for you to find the most common remedy that will work for your situation, right now, to help you achieve balance and healing.

- Regarding the homeopathic remedies included, or not included, in this book: As stated above, this is not a comprehensive study of homeopathy. Rather, this book is designed to give you information quickly and simply. I have included the top homeopathic remedies used by most practitioners, and the most popular conditions found in my daily practice.

- There are a few remedies presented as possible helps in the Condition Repertory chapter that do not appear in the Materia

Medica chapter. They are not as common, so you can look online or in a more comprehensive work for the keynotes, symptoms, modalities, etc. Likewise, there are a few remedies contained in the Materia Medica chapter that are not included in the Conditions chapter. These remedies are very common, but not connected to any conditions in this book. They will all be starred with an asterisk (*).

CHAPTER 1

Homeopathy Made Simple: What It Is, How To Use It

Having seen more than ten thousand clients in my practice so far, I'm excited to share their successes with you, so you can feel confident in using homeopathy as part of your healthcare regimen. Let's learn about homeopathy—what it is and how to use it. In this section you will discover:

- What homeopathy is, and how it began with the brilliant Dr. Samuel Hahnemann

- Three Principles of Homeopathy:

  1. Like cures like—the Law of Similars.

  2. The more a remedy is diluted, the greater its potency—the Law of the Infinitesimal Dose.

  3. Illness is specific to the individual (a holistic or whole-person approach).

- How to use homeopathy—how to find the right remedy; take and care for your homeopathic remedies; and make your own combination remedies

WHAT IS HOMEOPATHY?

Homeopathy is a traditional system of medicine that treats people's sufferings with very small, or minute, doses of a natural substances (from plants, minerals, etc.). It is a system of medicine used by hundreds of millions of people worldwide. Homeopathics are the most effective medicines that treat a wide range of conditions and diseases, offering vast healing possibilities in natural, low-cost, non-toxic remedies that can be taken by anyone—young or old, those who are pregnant or nursing, or those currently using over-the-counter or prescription medications. This natural medicine is a useful method of self-care for minor conditions, such as the common cold and flu.

The World Health Organization cited that homeopathic medicine should be used alongside conventional medicine in order to provide adequate global healthcare. From the beginning of the reign of Queen Victoria to the present day, the Royal Family of Britain has always had homeopaths as their personal physicians. Medical professionals in many countries use homeopathic medicine first in their practices. Most pharmacists in Europe dispense herbs and homeopathics, as well as conventional medications.

While my daughter was on her senior trip to Europe, in Rome she became a feast for the mosquitos, with multiple bites. She suffered much swelling and itching. After taking a conventional medication for allergic reactions (Benadryl), for twenty-four hours there was no relief. It was making her sleepy and dopey. She called me, crying. I suggested she visit a nearby pharmacy to pick up some Apis Mellifica. She went quickly and was surprised to find both homeopathic and conventional medicines in the pharmacy together. She felt better within hours, and to her joy, no sleepiness or feeling dopey! She was so happy to join her group again in their fun activities.

The FDA has determined that homeopathic remedies are safe to give a person in any condition. Homeopathy hasn't caused a fatality in over 200 years of use. These remedies will not interact with medications, yet, they can work to normalize healthy functioning of the body. They can cause no harm, even if a child were to open a bottle and eat all of the tasty sugar pellets. This is in contrast to the toxicity of prescription and over-the-counter medications. When my brother was a child, he ate a bottle of flavored aspirin and had to have his stomach pumped, or he would have died.

There are an estimated 160,000 to 300,000 deaths a year, in the United States alone, due to medications (either wrong type, or over-prescribed, or wrongly taken). Another disturbing fact with conventional medicines: seven classes of medications cause cognitive decline, Dementia, or brain-fog-like symptoms, among even more severe side effects. In addition to these frightening numbers, there are over 100,000 emergency room visits a year (in U.S. hospitals) due to prescription medications.

Many people visit homeopathic practitioners after spending vast amounts of money with conventional medicine and not getting favorable results. Or, because they need help with symptoms caused by prescribed medications. Still others desire to be free of doctor-prescribed medications, treatments, and their side effects. Homeopaths seek to treat the whole person rather than treating symptoms, thereby creating more longlasting results. However, we do *use* symptoms to find the right remedy.

Using homeopathic medicine, a person can re-establish balance and return to a healthier state. Health is feeling physically good and able, mentally feeling clear and making good decisions, and emotionally/spiritually feeling peaceful and calm inside.

If you select the right remedy, you may notice a change in your symptoms within minutes or hours for ailments that came on suddenly (acute). However, it may take days or weeks to notice a difference in longstanding (chronic) ailments. Homeopathic remedies are particularly effective in treating chronic illnesses that fail to respond to conventional treatment. They are also invaluable in helping with emotional and mental issues.

Homeopathic medicines are often used with other natural treatments such as herbs, flower essences and sometimes with essential oils. Always check the precautions of using different treatments together. Normally, natural remedies will not interact with each other, especially homeopathics. There has never been a death caused by the use of homeopathy. It is theoretically impossible.

How Homeopathy Began: Brilliant Dr. Hahnemann

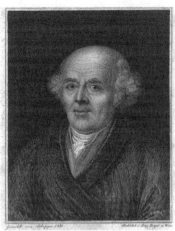

Homeopathy was founded by the celebrated German physician Samuel Hahnemann in the late eighteenth century. He was known for his work in pharmacology, hygiene, public health, industrial toxicology, and psychiatry. Also, he was a brilliant researcher and translator, transcribing medical writings into different languages (he spoke several). Reacting to the barbarous practices of his day, such as using leeches for bloodletting and toxic mercury-based laxatives, Dr. Hahnemann set out to find a more humane approach to medicine.

His breakthrough came while translating a particular medical document. He came across information about an herb called Cinchona (Peruvian Bark). It was high in quinine and had the ability to "cure" malaria. It intrigued him, so he formulated an experiment. He obtained the herb, which was quite toxic, and ingested it in a tea, twice daily. Soon, he developed a periodic fever common to malaria, as well as other symptoms. Then, as soon as he stopped taking the tea, his symptoms went away. His discovery was this: If taking a large dose of Cinchona created symptoms of malaria in a healthy person, this same substance—given to a sickly person in a smaller dose—might rouse the body to fight the disease. His theory was born out by many years of experiments with hundreds of substances, and analysis of the similar results they produced in humans. See his Principles of Homeopathy below.

He experimented with many substances that are still used to this day. They come from plants, minerals, drugs, disease products and animal parts. Hahnemann, in his medicines, used smaller and smaller doses. He would dilute the substance while using succussion (shaking) to create a remedy or medicine (see Principle 2, below: the Law of Infinitesimal

Dose). This is called "potentizing," so you will see a number with the homeopathic remedy name to signify how diluted it is. Using roman numerals, a 6X has been diluted six times to the tenth portion, a 6C has been diluted six times to the hundredth, a 1M has been diluted one time to the thousandth; more on potencies later in this chapter. After several dilutions, there is no toxicity, and after twenty-four dilutions, there is none of the original substance left.

> EXAMPLE OF A HOMEOPATHIC MEDICINE: A common remedy, or "polychrest" as it is called because it has so many uses, is Arsenicum Album. In any quantity, arsenic can make a person sick or even lead to death. But in minute doses, Arsenicum Album can abate symptoms of food poisoning, flu, burning symptoms, and more.

Some researchers think that homeopathic remedies work by some sort of electrical resonance, affecting our immune system, which is designed to restore order. The more similar the remedy is to the patient's symptoms, the closer the patient would come to "cure" or a return to health (Principle 1: the Law of Similars).

As Dr. Hahnemann learned more by making medicines, he tested them on human beings (humanely) in evaluations called "provings." During the proving process, a specific medicine was given to healthy volunteers, and their resulting symptoms were compiled by observers into a "matching symptom picture." Volunteers were observed for months at a time and made to keep extensive journals detailing all their own symptoms at specific times throughout the day. They were forbidden from consuming coffee, tea, spices, or wine for the duration of the experiment; playing chess was also prohibited because Dr. Hahnemann considered it to be "too exciting," although they *were* allowed to drink beer and encouraged to exercise in moderation. After the provings were completed, Hahnemann made each volunteer take an oath, swearing that what they reported in their journal was the truth. Then, he would interrogate them extensively concerning the symptoms they had recorded.

Through his great discovery of homeopathy, Dr. Hahnemann attracted students from all over Europe to Germany where he lived until the latter part of his life. He moved to Paris in the 1830s and was one of the most celebrated doctors of his time. He left volumes of records and books and trained many doctors in the art of homeopathy.

First, a book called a "repertory" (exact symptoms, accompanied by a small or large list of related homeopathic remedies) was made. A myriad of symptoms and their related remedies were compiled from all these provings that had been done. This is where the wisdom and experience of homeopathic practitioners has been collected for more than the past two hundred years. This medical repertory then became like an index to many homeopathic remedies that could be used for specific symptoms.

After this, a Materia Medica (or remedy guide) was created to allow the homeopath to see all the symptoms of each single remedy. In homeopathy you find the right remedy based upon your symptoms using the repertory, then by looking to the

> ### GUMS—TEETH
>
> **Bleeding easily**—Agave; *Alum.;* Ant. c.; *Arg. n.;* Ars.; Bor.; *Carbo v.;* Echin.; Iod.; *Kreos.;* Lach.; *Merc.; Nit. ac.; Phos.;* Plant.; Sul. ac.; Zinc.
> **Bleeding protractedly, after tooth extraction**—*Ham.;* Kreos.; Trill.
> **Blue line along margin of**—Plumb.
> **Burning of**—Antipyr. See Pain.
> **Cold feeling of**—Coccinel.
> **GUMBOIL—Inflammation of:** *Acon.;* Bell.; Bor.; Calc. fl.; Cham.; *Hekla;* Kreos.; *Merc.;* Phos.; Sil. See Pain, Swelling.
> **Painful, sore, sensitive**—Alum.; Arg. n.; *Bapt.;* Carbo v.; *Cham.; Hep.;* Kreos.; *Merc.;* Rhus t.; Sil.; Sul.; Thuya.
> **STROPHULUS—Red seam on:** *Ant. c.;* Apis; *Cham.;* Kali p.; Puls.; Rhus t.
> **Scorbutic (soft, spongy, receding)**—*Agave;* Ant. c.; Ars.; Bapt.; *Carbo. v.;* Echin.; Iod.; Kali c.; *Kreos.; Merc.;* Mur. ac.; Nat. m.; *Nit. ac.;* Phos.; Thuya.
> **Swelling of**—*Apis; Cham.;* Cistus; Lach.; Mag. m.; Merc. d.; *Merc. i. r.;* Mur. ac.; Phos.; Plumb.; Sul.
> **PYORRHŒA ALVEOLARIS—Ulceration of:** Aur.; *Bapt.;* Carbo v.; Caust.; *Cistus;* Kali c.; Kreos.; Merc. c.; *Nit. ac.;* Phos.; Sil.; Staph.

Public Doman. Source: Google Books. Pocket Manual of Homoeopathic Materia Medica: Comprising the Characteristic ... - William Boericke

Materia Medica to see how closely the remedy matches your situation.

THREE PRINCIPLES OF HOMEOPATHY

Based on his work, Dr. Hahnemann formulated the following Principles of Homeopathy, as we've noted above:

1. Like cures like—Law of Similars

2. The more a remedy is diluted, the greater its potency—Law of the Infinitesimal Dose

3. Illness is specific to the individual (a holistic or whole-person approach)

1. **Like cures like—Law of Similars**

According to Dr. Hahnemann, "Each individual case of disease is most surely, radically, rapidly, and permanently annihilated and removed only by a medicine capable of producing (in the human system) the most similar and complete manner of the totality of the symptoms." In other words, the same substance that in large doses produces the symptoms of illness, in very minute doses cures it. The word homeopathy is derived from the Greek words (*homoios*) for like or similar to, and (*patheia*) suffering, disease, or feeling. He referred to this phenomenon as the Law of Similars, a principle first recognized in the fourth century B.C.E. by Hippocrates, who was studying the effects of herbs upon disease. This Law of Similars was also the theoretical basis for the creation of vaccines by physicians Edward Jenner, Jonas Salk, and Louis Pasteur. They would "immunize" the body with trace amounts of a disease component, often a virus, to strengthen its immune response to the actual disease. Allergies are treated in a similar fashion today, by introducing minute quantities of the suspected allergen into the body to bolster natural tolerance levels.

2. **The more diluted, the greater its potency—Law of the Infinitesimal Dose**

Most people believe that the higher the dose of a medicine, the greater its effect. But the opposite holds true in homeopathy, where the more a substance is diluted, the higher its potency. Dr. Hahnemann realized the Law of the Infinitesimal Dose by experimenting with higher and higher dilutions of substances to avoid toxic side effects.

Today, homeopathic remedies are usually prepared through a process of diluting the original material (plants, minerals, etc.) with pure water or alcohol and succussing (vigorous shaking). Succussion is the key—it transfers the energy of the material into the molecules of the water or alcohol solution. Homeopathic solutions can be diluted to such an extent that literally no molecules of the original substance remain in the remedy. In fact, any homeopathic remedy over 24X potency (24 successive dilutions and succussions) will have no chemical trace of the original substance remaining. Thus, more succussions and dilutions equal a higher potency.

So, the more dilute it gets the more potent it becomes. This has been the source of great fascination among practitioners and researchers in the field of homeopathic medicine, from the conventional chemistry point of view; how can something work if there is no trace of the original substance? Most homeopaths believe that the original material or substance's energy signature (remember, like-cures-like) may signal the immune system to rebalance or initiate harmony where healing can take place.

3. Illness is specific to the individual

In explaining that illness is specific to the individual, a headache is not just a headache, it is unique to each person. For instance, you may suffer from chronic headaches, perhaps migraines. Consulting with a homeopathic practitioner is very different from in seeing a doctor of conventional medicine. While the conventional medical treatment for most headaches is the same for everyone (some form of analgesic or anti-inflammatory), homeopathy recognizes over two hundred symptom patterns associated with headaches and has corresponding remedies for each.

Your headache may be in the front of your head. It may get worse with a cold breeze, improve with heat, and come on during the morning; it may feel better while you are laying down, or while you are sitting up. Each of these is considered, as well as your constitution—you may be a person who is thin, easily excited, or the docile sedentary type. The main task of the homeopathic practitioner is a process called "taking the case" or recording all of the qualities—physical, mental, and emotional—that will determine the best remedy match for the patient.

Homeopaths consult vast compendiums of repertories (symptoms and the many remedies useful) and Materia Medicas (individual remedy symptom pictures) to determine the remedy that most closely matches the total picture of your symptoms. For instance, one would use a repertory to look for a compilation of those medicines that are specific for headaches that occur in the front of the head in the morning (in the "head" section, under the subsection "pain," under the further subsection "frontal pain worse in the morning").

After reviewing a person's various symptoms in the repertory, homeopaths go to the Materia Medica to see how each of the top remedies matches with the totality of your symptoms. A repertory and a Materia Medica complement each other. Remember these records have been used and updated through the past several hundred years; they contain hundreds of remedies, one of which matches your type of headaches most closely, and the way your body manifests symptoms. If you wish to study homeopathy further, I would suggest you purchase these guides.

Seeking individual care through "constitutional prescribing" by a homeopath can produce profound personal changes and even alter a person's, or their family's, life trajectory. Your constitution is the sum total of your physical, mental and emotional/spiritual symptoms or condition, how you handle life in general, and how you react to stresses in the environment, including relationships. There can be many layers to a person's health, so a constitutional prescription is best left to an experienced homeopath.

For example, a person may have rheumatoid arthritis, but is presenting to their homeopath the symptoms of a Phosphorus constitution, such as frequent nose bleeds, social skills, and an intuitive personality. The client may want to work on their arthritis, but the professional homeopath must determine the strategy to improve their overall health or constitution, and also be able to effectively deal with what the client wishes.

This book is more introductory and *condition* based—not constitution based—so you will gain the ability to use the most common homeopathic remedies for your family members' health. See a homeopath to find your *constitutional* remedy, and talk with them about possible layers that are presenting.

HOW TO USE HOMEOPATHY

Homeopathic medicines are identified by their Latin names. They come in many forms—liquid or dry, in pellets or tablets, creams or gels. In this section you will learn:

- How to find the right homeopathic remedy—the most similar to your symptoms

- Which potency to use—for acute, chronic, emergency, or emotional needs

- How to take homeopathic remedies—whether in pellets, liquid, or creams for skin

- Care for homeopathic remedies

- How to use or make homeopathic combinations

Let's make this simple. With the information in this book you may have the opportunity, within the next few years, to use over a hundred homeopathic remedies for many different health situations. You can buy remedies from your local health-food store as you need them, or you may choose to acquire a kit of remedies, which is much more economical than buying them individually.

Kits come in different potencies. I have a 30C kit that has a hundred remedies. These work for most of my needs, and my clients' needs as well. Add more remedies for specialized health conditions that you encounter.

Some people use higher potencies, such as 200C and 1M, or higher, but I would generally leave that to professionals. 200C potencies are important for emergencies, and can also help emotional issues when the professional is using the remedy that matches a client's symptoms most closely. But some sensitive people may react poorly to them (and certainly we don't want to do more harm than good). Remember, low potencies and simple keynotes often win the race, like the tortoise passing the hare.

How to Find the Right Homeopathic Remedy

The more similar the remedy is to your symptoms (Homeopathic Principle 1), the more prompt should be the return to health. Selecting the correct remedy, you may notice a change in symptoms within minutes or hours for an ailment that came on quickly. Often, I have seen many clients get quick results. It may take days or weeks to notice a difference in chronic ailments. In my practice, however, I have repeatedly seen homeopathic remedies help in chronic illnesses that had failed to respond to conventional medical treatment.

In this book, there are a few ways to find a remedy most similar to your symptoms. First, go to Chapter 2 to find the condition and symptoms you may be experiencing. Once you locate your condition/symptoms, you will see several of the top remedies recommended for that condition. Conditions are listed alphabetically at the top of each page. Read through some of their descriptions to see if any seem to match. Settle on one or two.

Then go to Chapter 3 (Materia Medica) to find the homeopathic remedy or remedies you've chosen and to get additional details. See if the Keynotes match; see if the Physical or Mental/Emotional symptoms match; see if the Modalities match, and so on. You may find only one remedy that is close enough, or that several remedies would apply.

If you can't get a match that you feel comfortable with, try the one that's the closest fit anyway, in a 30C or lower potency. If totally confused, try using three or four of the top remedies in a combination (see Using and Making Combinations Below). *All* your symptoms do not need to match all the symptoms of one remedy in order for the remedy to affect change and bring healing. For our purposes here, you should feel confident in being able to use the remedy closest to your symptoms. You may also study another Materia Medica or medical repertory, or other homeopathic books, or seek out the services of a homeopathic practitioner in your area or online.

NOW, TRY IT—A PRACTICE SESSION

Example: Susan has a minor injury with bruising and soft tissue damage (no bones involved). Do the following:

- Go to Chapter 2 (pp. 19-135) and find the page or pages that deal with Injuries (pp. 87-89). Conditions are listed alphabetically, like a dictionary, with names of Condtions on the top of each page. You can also check the Table of Contents, and find Chapter 2, Injuries, p. 87.

- The remedy seems to be **Arnica** because it says it's first in all injuries and specific for soft injuries.

- Next go to Chapter 3, and check alphabetical listing at the top of each page to find Arnica, in this case p.149. Notice that the **KEYNOTES** include its uses—first in injuries, shock, bruising, overtraining. Check physical symptoms. Seems to fit well.

Note: There are a few remedies presented in the Conditions chapter (Chapter 2) that do not appear in the Materia Medica chapter (Chapter 3), like Drosera for Bronchitis, for example. These remedies are omitted here as they are not as common. They will be starred with an asterisk (*) in the Conditions chapter.

Other ways to find remedies: look in the Quick Reference (Chapter 4) for guides to top remedies, top keynotes, and to find mention of the specific "something" that is bothering you the most or, as we call it, "presenting itself."

Which Potency to Use

Many people ask, "What potency do I take?" when they find a single remedy right for their circumstances. Potency relates to how dilute the remedy is. It is, however, more important to have the right remedy than the right potency. Any potency will do. If it is the right remedy it will be helpful enough to bring the immune system or vital energy into greater balance, so that the body can help itself.

As we learned in Homeopathy Principle 2, the more a substance is diluted, the higher its potency. There is a wide range of thought about using potencies. Low potencies such as 6X or 6C are generally used in commercial formulas as these address very physical symptoms, such as flu aches, allergies, or digestive gas symptoms, etc. I will usually suggest

30X and 30C potencies which work for most situations because they can treat physical and/or emotional issues with great success. 200C potencies are reserved mostly for emergency situations like injuries, or for deeper long-standing emotional issues. 200C and 1M or high potencies should generally (and ideally) be used when under the care of a skilled homeopathic practitioner.

In my experience and homeopathic practice, I apply the following **three patterns** for using different potencies. And I always start at low potencies and go higher as needed.

1. For **acute** (recent) and **chronic** (longstanding) conditions, use 6X, 6C, 30X, or 30C potencies, and take two pellets, three times a day. I use these potencies because they are most available from companies like Boiron, Hylands (Standard), and Washington.

2. In **emergency**, like injuries or burns, and as noted previously, I recommend the use of the higher potency of 200C, two pellets several times a day as needed, reducing the frequency as symptoms improve. I find that mild to medium pain levels do well with 30C or 200C, used several times a day. Higher pain levels, use 200C several times an hour until pain subsides. Note: the sooner you use a remedy after the injury, the faster the results (pain goes away quicker).

3. Using homeopathic remedies for **emotional symptoms** requires a clear homeopathic symptom picture or cause. Because it will work more deeply, use a 200C potency, two pellets once a week. The person should see positive results within a couple of weeks or so.

How to Take Homeopathic Remedies

Homeopathic medicines are different from conventional medications. Conventionally, if you want a stronger effect out of an aspirin, most people take more than one. With homeopathy, if you want a stronger effect, take it *more often*. Remember, more is not always better, but more often may be the key to success. The homeopathic remedy works best as it matches your symptoms closely. Stop using the remedy as the symptoms go away. You may safely take a remedy every few minutes in a crisis.

Homeopathic remedies come in different varieties: orals in dry (pellets or tablets), or using pellets in water, liquid (prepared drops), and topicals to use on skin (creams or gels). One dose is usually a couple of tablets, or a few pellets dissolved under the tongue, or a few liquid drops held under the tongue. Topicals are applied to the skin in the affected area of bruising, pain, or wound. Use homeopathic remedies as follows:

- **Dry (pellets or tablets).** Pellets come in sucrose, or tablets in pressed lactose. Gently pour 2-3 pellets into the lid of the container, then drop the pellets into your mouth from the cap, and place under your tongue (avoid touching the pellets with your hands). Let them dissolve and or chew them. Some tablets come in pillow packs and just need to be popped out. If you are using more than one remedy you may take them at the same time, however it is better that you not open more than one bottle at a time. Under normal circumstances, take lower potencies, like 30C, two or three times a day. Pellets may also be placed in water, stirred and dissolved, and then sipped throughout the day. Different potencies call for different intervals of time in between doses. Take the remedy until the symptoms change.

- **Liquid (prepared drops).** Take the number of drops indicated on the bottle, unless otherwise directed. Place drops directly under the tongue and retain there for at least 30 seconds. Avoid touching any part of the dropper to the mouth or tongue. If you are using more than one remedy you may take them at the same time.

- **Topicals (creams, gels).** Most topical creams or gels should be used on the skin several times a day. Many people like gels because they dry quickly so clothing won't stick. In my experience, creams are preferred because I feel they release the medicine over a longer period of time so they go deeper and last longer.

A note before taking homeopathic remedies: Make the most of your remedies. It is best not to brush teeth, eat or drink anything for at least 10 minutes before or after administration of the remedy. Also, do not use gum, mints, or toothpaste containing any mint within 30 minutes of taking a remedy. CAUTION: It is best to refrain from using products containing camphor, menthol, or strong essential oils. But if you need to use them, in my experience homeopathic remedies can be taken at least 2 hours before or after them.

If you are using prescription or over-the-counter medications: Many of my clients come into our consultations with lists of medications their doctor has prescribed for them. Since this is such a common occurrence, and with so many people using use over-the-counter and prescription drugs, my advice is, "Don't stop any medication without your doctor's advice. *Never* go off prescription drugs without consulting your healthcare professional. It may be dangerous or life-threatening.

Most doctors will help you to reduce the dose of prescription medication, if you can show them your health is improving. I also ask my clients how well their medication is working for them. Interestingly, some say it makes all the difference, others are not as pleased. It all depends on the medication and the disease as to how fast one can reduce and come off them. In general, taking homeopathic remedies will not interfere or react with a person's medication.

Care for Homeopathic Remedies

Take care of your homeopathic remedies. When taking homeopathic pellets, avoid touching the pellets with your hands. Keep all homeopathic remedies out of direct sunlight. Store them three feet away from a microwave oven, computer, or television set. Keep them away from strong odors such as mint, essential oils, menthol or camphor (as discussed above). It is not necessary to refrigerate.

Using or Making Homeopathic Combinations

If you want to use more than a single remedy at a time, you can buy or make your own combination. Homeopathic combinations account for a large portion of the homeopathic remedies sold. Combinations are packaged in the name of a condition or ailment such as "Sore Throat" or "Allergies." They generally contain 2C to 30C potencies and offer good results when the symptom picture or simillimum is not altogether clear. Adults and children, even animals, respond well to them. Use them as directed on the package or bottle.

Some people assert that "combinations work because the body uses parts of the remedies it needs." Others will say, "the body chooses the right remedy from the combination, and tends to ignore the rest." Use combinations prepared by reputable companies, or make your own with the low-potency (2C-30C) homeopathics you have on hand.

You can make your own combination by using a few of the remedies listed in the Conditions chapter (2), for your particular situation. In generally, I like to include up to five or six homeopathic remedies in a formula, yet two or three are just fine. To make your own combination, put one pellet of each remedy in a small dropper bottle. Fill halfway with purified water and let the pellets dissolve. Fill the bottle with alcohol (EverClear). Succuss, or shake, several times. This will last for a couple of weeks in the fridge. Take three drops three times a day.

If you want to look up more remedies for your condition, using a homeopathic repertory such as *Robin Murphy's Medical Repertory*, it will show the most popular homeopathic remedies in a particular group of symptoms. In Murphy's Repertory the remedies in **extra-bold type** are likely candidates for a combination. Even better, some symptoms have **EXTRA-BOLD CAPITAL LETTERS**—these remedies are called the "leaders of the group." They will work even better for a truly good combination.

USE OF UPPER CASE IN THIS BOOK:

UPPER CASE in the following chapters indicates a "defining action," that is, a primary symptom or indicator.

HEALING THROUGH HOMEOPAPTHY

In healing with homeopathy, all that is required is to find the right remedy; take it, and it will change things. It's like peeling an onion, one layer at a time. What is presenting right now? What has been there for a long time? Your homeopath can help you in discerning the priority. Admittedly, there are some things too deep to resolve with just homeopathy; in this book we are talking about healing common health issues. So, in homeopathy when using the right remedy, the body will correct itself and the condition will resolve. You don't need to continue taking the remedy. Acute or chronic issues will have different expected healing times. This type of healing is desirable, unlike taking Western medications where many people are told they will have to stay on their medications for life. It not only creates dependency or possible economic hardship, but also side effects that can further damage a person's health.

Aggravations

You might wonder about side effects from homeopathic medicines. There can be! They are called "aggravations" and happen infrequently. However, they are not creating dependence, economic hardship, or damage to a person's health. Rather they are part of healing. Generally speaking, when a homeopathic remedy causes a condition to grow worse, an aggravation may be taking place. It is important to understand two types of aggravation:

- First, a healing aggravation occurs where the body is working to push out old symptoms (deep stuff) trying to create balance, which makes the condition worse for a day or two, then things get better permanently

- The other type of aggravation happens when a client is over-enthusiastic while taking a high potency (200C or higher) and uses it too often. This can bring on an aggravation as well. In practice, I rarely see aggravations, especially when using the lower potencies of 6X to 30C.

Provings

Now that we have talked about aggravations, we need to talk about proving—namely, testing and reporting on the results of a remedy you are taking. Can you prove a remedy? Yes. Occasionally, someone could be using the wrong remedy in a high potency for some time, and "prove" the symptoms of that remedy. Or, rarely, a very sensitive person could take on the symptoms of the homeopathic remedy they are taking, and mimic them. If this happens, simply quit taking the remedy, and if you are taking a low potency the symptoms will go away in just a few hours (high potency may take more time). Remember, these things are quite rare.

If you wish to, find a homeopath you can trust who will help you navigate the healing process. On your own, in moving forward all you need to do is to try, experiment, and be patient. Soon, you will be writing your own success stories with homeopathy.

CHAPTER 2

Conditions

This chapter contains detailed descriptions and suggested remedies for each of the conditions listed below. The descriptions and remedies will follow (in section II. CONDITIONS REPERTORY) in alphabetical order.

I. HEAD TO TOE

EMOTIONAL
Anxiety
Depression
Grief

HEAD
Head injuries

EYES
Conjunctivitis
Hay fever
Macular degeneration
Vision problems

EARS
Earaches

FACE
Acne

NOSE
Hay fever
Mucus
Nose bleeds
Sinus

MOUTH
Canker sores
Cold sores
Sore throat
Teething
Toothaches

NECK
Acne
Sore throat

NERVOUS SYSTEM
Nerve pain
Sciatica
Shingles
Tremors

BACK
Acne
Back pain

CHEST/LUNGS
Bronchitis
Cough
Palpitations
Pneumonia

ARMS/HANDS
Gout
Sweating (under arms)
Warts

JOINTS
Arthritis

ABDOMEN/DIGESTIVE
Bloating
Colic in babies
Gallstones
Gas
Heartburn
Morning sickness

URINARY
Bedwetting
Incontinence
Urinary tract infection

FEMALE
Hot flashes
Menopause
Menstrual issues
Morning sickness
PMS

MALE
Prostate

CHILDREN
Bed wetting
Colic in babies
Diaper rash
Teething

LOWER ABDOMEN
Constipation
Diaper rash
Diarrhea
Hemorrhoids

LEGS
Leg ulcers
Varicose veins

FEET
Gout

SKIN
Abscesses/boils
Acne
Bites and stings
Bruising
Burns
Eczema
Itching
Psoriasis
Warts

MECHANICAL
Injuries
Muscle cramps

ILLNESS
Fevers
Flu
Mononucleosis

CONDITIONS

Exhaustion	Obesity
Gout	Shingles
Hay fever	Travel sickness
Hypoglycemia	Tremors

II. CONDITIONS REPERTORY: MATCH YOUR SYMPTOMS, FIND A REMEDY

This chapter is your Repertory. From skin issues to toothaches, heartburn to shingles, back pain to flu, we all experience bumps and bruises, and illness in life. Using your symptoms, the first book a homeopath will reference is a Medical Repertory (an inventory of symptoms and their related usable remedies listed) This is called "reportizing." It will lead them to the specific remedy that matches your symptoms the most.

The repertory here is a little different. These are the most common conditions for which clients come to see me. Also, with each condition you will find a brief description of common symptoms, client success stories, and some of my general experiences. Then, the remedies offered here are not just the most frequently used in homeopathy, but also the most popular in my practice. It should be easy for you to choose one, or more if needed.

Here's how to find the remedy:

1. Find your condition, listed here in alphabetical order.
   What is affecting your health the most right now? Try to only work on one thing at a time.

2. Match your symptoms.
   Look through the remedies listed to find one with symptoms that match yours (the more similar, the better). As noted, in the following chapters, UPPER CASE will indicate a "defining action," that is, a primary symptoms.

3. Choose the remedy.
   Once you have found symptoms that match yours in a remedy or two, go to Chapter 3, to compare them in more detail, then

choose one. Keep it simple. But, if there's more than one remedy that fits your situation, that's okay. Make a combination (see
Chapter 1: Using and Making Homeopathic Combinations).

4. Take the remedy.
    Follow guidelines in Chapter 1 on how to take homeopathic
    remedies and what potency to use.

Homeopathy is a great tool to use in healing. Why not try it first,
rather than using other medications which cause side effects? Now,
always remember that injuries (page 87) should always be treated first.
And, if you have any questions about what to do next, refer to "How to
Use this Book" in the introduction. Go, find your remedy.

The conditions noted in Section I (Head to Toe) are described next,
listed in alphabetical order. Like a dictionary format, check at top of
each page to quickly find your condition.

ABSCESSES/BOILS

Abscesses are bacterial infections that the body has walled-off, created pus around and enclosed. The body will eventually reabsorb it, or it will erupt (break out). Abscesses are more open wounds whereas boils are more like a volcano waiting to erupt. Abscesses, or boils, start with a poor immune system, or an injury that deposits bacteria that will fester. Poor diet and lifestyle contribute to poor immunity.

Abscess Story

A woman came to me complaining of a wound in her thigh bone which involved a piece of wood and it would abscess frequently. It had been there for over thirty years. Every six weeks it created a great deal of pus, erupted, and then would heal over. I suggested she try Silicea. She began using the remedy. About a week later, her wound created a large amount of pus that erupted again, but this time what came out of the wound was surprising. She was able to remove a piece of wood the size of 1/8 inch x 1/2 inch, with her fingers. It finally healed up for good and hasn't bothered her since.

Abscesses/Boils Essential Remedies

Top 3 remedies:

Calc Sulph—#1 REMEDY FOR ABSCESSES/BOILS.[1] Acne with pus, pus easily, yellow pus in crusts, scabs, or discharges. Helps to ripen (erupt) or re-absorb abscesses and boils. Better with local heat.

Hepar Sulph—any injury which causes pus. Chronic rashes. Stinging, burning. Deep cracks. Better from pressure, worse from touch. Sensitive to draft. INFECTIONS.

Silicea—skin can pus easily, scars easily. Impetigo. Brittle nails. Smelly feet. THIN, COLD PEOPLE. Expels foreign objects, i.e. splinters.

---

[1] As noted previously, use of UPPER CASE indicates a "defining action," that is, a primary symptom.

Other important remedies:

Arnica—bruising. After injuries. Marbled skin. Crops of small boils. Bed sores. Petechiae (red spots). Tingling. Itching that moves around.

Lachesis—skin bluish, PURPLE APPEARANCE. Cellulitis. Burning ulcers. Bed sores with black edges. Scars break open and bleed. Worse on the left side.

Mercury Sol or Mercury Viv—bleeding gums. Moist skin. Itches. Ulcers. Cutting pains. Itching, yellow jaundice skin. Moist eczema. Everything worse from warmth of bed. Worse draft, getting cold, and at night.

Abscesses/Boils most important for size, pus discharge, resolving types.

Size		Pus discharge		Resolving types	
Large:	Hepar Sulph Lachesis Merc Sol Silicea	**Bad smelling:**	Hepar Sulph Lachesis Merc Sol Arnica Silicea	**Ripening-erupting:**	Hepar Sulph Silicea Merc Sol
Small:	Arnica	**Yellow-green:**	Calc Sulph Hepar Sulph Merc Sol Silicea	**Re-absorbing:**	Calc Sulph Lachesis Silicea Arnica
		Bloody:	Hepar Sulph Merc Sol Silicea Arnica Lachesis		

ACNE

Acne is an excess of sebum, which is an oil that supports skin moisture and integrity. Excess sebum plugs pores and can create acne, or blackheads. Acne generally comes from hormonal imbalances, male or female. The liver becomes overburdened and can't detoxify the body, so toxins find another way out—through the skin. It is aggravated by a poor diet, including bad fats and excess sugars. Constipation and hemorrhoids may be present, and are also associated with liver health. Change your diet and use homeopathic remedies.

Acne Story
In my experience, healing acne is a gradual process and unique to each individual. There is no typical scenario, but it commonly goes away in one to two months. The healing mechanism is an internal thing, and progresses at its own pace. It's like turning a train—you can't turn a train on a dime. It takes a while for the body to reevaluate the chemistry inside, and balance itself again, taking time. If there is scarring with the acne, it can resolve, but will take an additional month or two. The scarring may require a different remedy—Silicea is good for scarring. If the body is acidic, it can make acne worse, but is more of a contributing factor, not the cause of the acne.

Acne Essential Remedies

Hepar Sulph—acne on forehead, lips, and in crops. Acne bleeds easily, is painful, sticking and prickling, or is sensitive to the touch. Acne has thick white discharge. Bloody acne with pus.

Kali Brom—acne on forehead, mouth, nose, shoulders, back. Acne is hard, blue or red, with scars. Itching acne. CYSTIC (boil-like) acne. Yellow pus. Hormone-related acne.

Nux Vomica—forehead acne that is red and blotchy, with constipation from laxative abuse. Worse consuming alcohol or cheese. Accompanied with irritability.

Rhus Tox—forehead acne, typically blister-like. Frequently accompanied by a red face, swelling. May be experiencing stiffness or arthritis.

Sepia—acne around the mouth and on the chin. #1 remedy when acne in young women is worse at menstruation. Craves sour taste. Constipation. Caused from low blood sugar (hypoglycemia), and nursing.

Silicea—cheek and forehead acne with PITTING SCARS or with pus that itch and burn. THIN, SHY, delicate people. Scars easily.

Sulphur—acne on nose with unhealthy-looking (dirty) skin. Skin smells bad (like rotten eggs). Worse heat, and at night.

Thuja—#1 remedy for acne in TEENAGE BOYS with greasy skin.

ADDICTIONS

Addictions are behaviors and cravings that start controlling one's life. These behaviors are compulsive, and interrupt the normal flow of life, and can disrupt relationships. The person will do almost anything to continue these addictive behaviors or drugs. Causation of addictions are usually some emotional trauma, but not always. The person is trying to reduce or numb their emotional pain by using drugs, alcohol, or adopting addictive behaviors. Western medicine uses prescription medications that suppress or disconnect a person from their emotions, and there may be many other side effects. Using homeopathy, even alongside prescription medications, can give one hope, and help to resolve these deep emotional issues.

Addiction Story
A successful businessman came to see me regarding a digestive issue. In our consultation, he also told me he drank seven to eight beers a day as well as using other stimulants. Apparently, he had no problems at home or work. I suggested the remedy Nux Vomica. Two weeks later, during

our consultation, he remarked that he felt better than he ever had, disclosing that he no longer had a desire for beer or other stimulants.

Addiction Essential Remedies

Aurum Met—addictions from having FINANCIAL PROBLEMS. Suicidal depression. Uses alcohol, opiates, craves stimulants. More masculine than feminine.

China/Cinchona—sensitive personality. Loss of fluids. Cravings for alcohol, beer, marijuana, cocaine, opiates, stimulants. Useful for hangovers.

Lachesis—addictive personality. Family history of addiction. Uses alcohol, opiates, stimulants. More feminine than masculine. OVER-TALKATIVE and vivacious. Can't stand things tight around their neck. Worse around menstruation. Remedy also used for Bipolar disorder.

Nux Vomica—BUSINESSMAN. Irritable person. Uses alcohol, beer, amphetamines, opiates, smoking tobacco. Useful for hangovers. Useful for withdrawal symptoms as well.

Sulphur—INTELLECTUAL, inventor type, more masculine than feminine. Alcohol, beer, marijuana, cocaine, opiates, stimulants. Weakness. Useful for withdrawal symptoms. Useful for hangovers.

ANXIETY

Anxiety is a sense of restlessness, which can go deeper into an indefinite uneasiness. Symptoms of anxiety often include sleeplessness, diarrhea, heart palpitations and even full-blown panic attacks. Causations of anxiety can range from hormonal imbalances to emotional traumas, family or work stresses, or trying to compensate for stress. Western medicine uses benzodiazepine drugs to treat anxiety, with their addictive qualities and sometimes severe mental side effects. Homeopathy shines in this realm as it can be taken alongside other medications. Matching the right homeopathic remedy to your symptoms can bring relief gradually, or sometimes even dramatically.

Anxiety Story
I met with a woman to discuss her digestive problems and her anxiousness. She was a piano performer. As we talked, her symptoms matched Argentum Nitricum, so she started using the remedy. She reported back in a couple of weeks that her digestion improved. She also revealed she had been suffering from performance anxiety and it too had improved greatly as well.

Anxiety Essential Remedies

Aconite—anxiety mainly from FRIGHT or shock. Anxiety and panic attacks worse in crowds, with severe palpitations.

Argentum Nit—performance anxiety. Severe anticipation, worse from crowds. #1 remedy for panic attacks. Nervousness. Crave sweets. Fears heights.

Arsenicum Album—PERFECTIONIST. Fears of health issues and death for self and family. Severe insecurities. Symptoms worse 10 P.M. to 2 A.M.

Gelsemium—anticipation anxiety. SHAKING. Panic attacks from shock, emotionally shuts down. Palpitations. Fears crowds.

Kali Arsenicosum—fear of heart disease or health issues. #2 remedy for panic attacks. Severe palpitations. Nervous. Worse in crowds.

Phosphorus—Nervous with palpitations. Panic attacks. EXTROVERT. Oversensitive people, empaths. Everything worse in crowds. History of nose bleeds.

ARTHRITIS

Arthritis is pain, inflammation, and sometimes deformation of joints; its symptoms can include mild aches and pains, to pain so severe that one can no longer function. There is gouty arthritis, osteoarthritis which is most common, rheumatoid arthritis, and psoriatic arthritis (osteoarthritis plus psoriasis). An inherited weakness, cold damp weather conditions, injuries, overuse, or poor diet, can bring on arthritis. Western medicine offers pain relievers (over-the-counter meds) that don't improve underlying conditions; these have been proven to damage the gastrointestinal system and more. Correctly chosen homeopathic remedies can help with underlying causes, leading the person to better overall health.

Arthritis Story

Many people come to me complaining of stiff joints and arthritic pain from weather changes. They are stiff when getting out of a chair, but are better from continued motion. Rhus Tox is the remedy that fits these symptoms. It tends to help a great many people. I have seen it help spinal injuries too. If this remedy doesn't work for you, seek a homeopath so they can take your case more carefully.

Arthritis Essential Remedies

Aconitum—arthritis from exposure to cold dry wind. Numbness and tingling. Lame, bruised, heavy, numb joints.

Apis Mel—SWELLING, stinging, red, swollen joints. Throbbing swollen joints. Better cold applications.

Belladonna—joints red and swollen, THROBBING. Cramping pain, cold, paralytic, weakness. Limping. Worse right side.

Bryonia—arthritis pain WORSE FROM MOTION. Sharp pain. Caused by injury or emotional trauma. Sprains. Joints red, swollen and hot. Liver involvement. Worse right side.

Kali Carb—arthritis caused by catching cold, or over-straining of joints. Deformation in small joints. Sharp aching pains. OBESITY. Worse from 2 to 4 AM.

Ledum—arthritis from injuries. Gouty arthritis. Nodules. Shooting pains, specifically in small joints.

Rhus Tox—#1 remedy for arthritis. Injuries, strains, cold damp conditions cause arthritis. Cracking joints. STIFFNESS better continued motion, worse change of weather. Better heat.

Silicea—arthritis in THIN, DELICATE, COLD PEOPLE. Caused by vaccinations, overworking joints, or cold. Loss of strength. Icy cold sweaty feet.

ASTHMA

Asthma is a breathing problem where there is difficulty breathing out. It happens occasionally with a cough, or when there is dust, pollen, or cold air. It starts with coughing and may only last a few minutes. If it lasts longer there may be a feeling of suffocation. Mucus production may happen. Asthma may be caused by emotional stress, grieving, and most commonly, inflammation caused by pollen, dust, cold air, or physical exertion. Western drugs used to treat asthma are usually steroid inhalers (that have toxicity and never get to the underlying cause). They also cause habituation (dependency).

Asthma Story

Asthma is a condition often treated with steroid inhalers, and only keeps the breathing under control while causing side effects. Most people are satisfied with their breathing when using these steroid inhalers. They are afraid to get off them, or afraid that natural medicines might react with their inhaler. I had a person come to me with asthma, who was very nervous and a perfectionist. Arsenicum album was the recommended remedy. Using Arsenicum 30C, daily, after two months made them feel considerably better. Their doctor reduced the steroid inhaler every two months and, eventually, they were off all medications and breathing well. Always consult your doctor. See Bronchitis condition as well.

Asthma Essential Remedies

Arsenicum album—acute or chronic uses. Wheezing and tightness of chest, worse from 10 P.M. to 2 A.M. Burning pains, must lie down or sit upright. Worse from cold. Extreme restlessness.

Kali Carb—mostly chronic asthma in obese individuals. Worse from 2 to 4 A.M. or waking. Anxiety, getting a cold causes asthma. Worse draft, motion, lying on the left side. Asthma alternates with nighttime diarrhea.

Lobelia—typically an acute or recent asthma. Feels hysterical, unable to breathe with WHEEZING. Feels like a lump in the chest. Feels worse with draft, cold or damp. Better from walking fast, slow deep breathing. Excessive amounts of mucus.

Cuprum Met—for recent and long-term asthma with VIOLENT SPASMS and a deep cough. The face turns blue. Worse generally nights and at 3 A.M. Caused by anger, fright, or other strong emotions. The thumbs are often clenched.

Ipecac—for recent and long-term asthma which has a rattling, SUFFOCATING cough, and face appears blue. Especially good for children. Coughs cause GAGGING and vomiting. Worse with dampness, lying down, motion, warmth or heat. Hands and feet are cold with sweating. Has cold ears. Lots of mucus.

Nat Sulph—for long-term asthma, effective for children and adults. Asthma worse 4 to 5 A.M., evening, especially when going to bed. Especially worse in damp weather, fog, storms, motion. It is allergic asthma. Often stops at puberty and will return in midlife. Rattling mucus in chest, can be green. Asthma with head injury.

BACK PAIN

Back pain is a common ailment in our society. There are many types of back pain as well as inflammation, redness, swelling, and pain that arises from movement or being at rest. Pain can also be affected by temperature, weather conditions, and time of day. Other symptoms include pinched nerves, as in sciatic pain. Western medicine treats back pain with mostly NSAIDs (non-steroidal anti-inflammatory drugs), and other medications—both with bad side effects. Chiropractors are often a helpful resource. Causes of back pain are usually some type of injury, slow degeneration, old age, or weather conditions. Homeopathic remedies can offer some relief or even amazing help.

Back Pain Story
I consulted with a man about his back pain. The pain was sharp and shooting in his lower back. He had previously consulted another homeopath who recommended Hypericum. He used Hypericum 30C and it worked quickly and perfectly on his pain, for five minutes at a time. Discouraged, he came to see me. Since Hypericum had helped, I suggested he take a higher dose, maybe a 200C potency. He did, and it worked for one hour. Then, he tried a 1M potency which worked for a whole day. Finally, he used a 10M potency one time. It permanently helped relieve the pain.

Back Pain Essential Remedies

Arnica—#1 remedy for First Aid, #1 remedy for injury, #1 remedy for soft tissue injury. Lumbar problems. Sciatica from injury. Stiffness, worse getting up from sitting. Worse from lying down, motion, and walking.

Bryonia—sharp pain. Sciatica SHARP and stabbing on motion. All pain WORSE FROM MOTION. Stiffness worse bending backwards, breathing, throbbing, lying down, motion, walking. Worse for women during menstruation. Mostly right-sided.

Calc Carb—thoracic (middle back) and lumbar (lower back) pain, worse getting up from sitting. Sciatica. Sharp pains. Hyperextended (overly mobile) joints, including weak ankles. OBESITY. Stiffness bending backwards. Back pain from injury, worse lying down, lifting, motion, sitting.

Lycopodium—Stiffness. Sharp pains worse evening, lying down, motion. Thoracic (middle back) and lumbar (lower back) pain. Burning right-sided sciatica, worse from sitting. Everything is worse sitting, walking, and from 4 to 8 P.M. Mostly in men with poor self-esteem.

Nat Mur—Thoracic (middle back), lumbar (lower back) pain. Sciatica, worse lying down. Worse getting up from sitting, Sharp pain, worse bending backwards, breathing, lying down, sitting. Stiffness. Back pain with depression, craves salt. Isolates self. HATES CONSOLATION.

Nux Vomica— Lumbar (lower back) pains, getting up from sitting. Sharp pains worse bending backwards. Stiffness worse breathing, evening, lying down, lifting, motion, sitting, walking. Sciatica worse motion, morning, night. Mostly males with POOR DIGESTION. Angry. Crave stimulants.

Rhus Tox—#1 remedy for back pain, #1 remedy for stiffness worse from first motion, better from continued motion. Back pain from injury. Sharp pains. Sciatica burning, worse from cold, at night, lying on the painful side. Worse before storms. Worse on waking, evenings, lying down, lifting, sitting, walking. BETTER FROM CONTINUED MOTION.

Sepia—Thoracic (middle back) and lumbar (lower back) pain. Sharp pains. Stiffness. Worse from bending back, breathing, evenings. Sciatica right sided, sitting. Throbbing pains worse from lifting, motion, sitting, walking. Mostly women with MENSTRUAL or MENOPAUSAL PROBLEMS. Intuitive. Isolative.

Sulphur—Thoracic (middle back) and lumbar (lower back) pain. Burning pains. Sharp pain. Stiffness. Sciatica burning, better with motion. Worse ascending, breathing, evenings, lying down, sitting, walking, before menstruation, and at night. Mostly MALE INTELLECTUALS with skin problems who are overheated.

BEDWETTING

Bedwetting occurs when children (commonly) or adults (not-so-commonly) urinate involuntarily at night. Under the age of five it is quite normal for a child to wet the bed (not normal when the child is older). Bedwetting is complex—the cause may come from kidney or bladder weakness, or an emotional reaction to family stresses, abuse, or fears.

Bedwetting Story
Many mothers ask what can be done for their child who wets the bed. The correctly chosen remedy can offer some results in one to four weeks, or for lasting results when taken longer. If not sure about just one remedy, using more than one remedy at a time is appropriate.

Bedwetting Essential Remedies

Argentum Nit—dreams of snakes or nightmares, fear of heights, PANIC ATTACKS, digestive issues. Sugar cravings.

Arsenicum album—anxious. Restless sleep. Twitching during sleep. Nightmares of death, dead people, water, misfortunes. Perfectionist. Organized and restless person. Worse 10 P.M. to 2 A.M.

Causticum—bedwetting during FIRST SLEEP. Moves legs, arms, and talks during the night. Worse 3 to 4 A.M. Incontinence. Concerned about injustice—"That's not fair" attitude.

Equisetum—#1 remedy for bedwetting when there are no other indications. Nightmares when passing urine, dreams of crowds of people. Pain in kidneys, constant urge to urinate. Frequent urination at night.

Kreosotum—child must be caressed before sleep (needs a story to go to sleep). Tosses about, laughs during sleep. Does not wake easily. Dreams of being pursued, of urination, or erections. Teething problems.

Lycopodium—cries at night. Laughs and cries during sleep. Dreams of sickness, or accidents. Hungry at night. Awaken terrified, unrested. Poor self-esteem. Bullied or is a bully. Meltdowns from 4 to 8 P.M.

Pulsatilla—bedwetting on first sleep. Talks, whines, screams during sleep. Anxious, disgusting dreams cause weeping. Mostly female, PEOPLE PLEASERS, weepy whiney, want to be held. Restless.

Sepia—bedwetting on first sleep. Dreams of being pursued, raped, urinating. Dreams worse lying on the left side. From family divorces. Mostly females.

BITES AND STINGS

Bites and stings manifest with redness, swelling, itching, pain, or destruction of tissue. Homeopathic remedies can help the body reduce itching, swelling and pain, deactivate toxins, support the liver, and repair damaged tissue. Homeopathic First-Aid can help symptoms quickly.

Bites and Stings Story

In casual conversation, my neighbor told me that she was sensitive to bee stings and always kept an EpiPen nearby. I shared my experiences of homeopathy with her and a remedy that might help her as well, and just as fast. The next week she was stung by a bee, and instead of using her EpiPen she tried Apis Mel 200C immediately. Her reaction to the sting subsided quickly. This is a common response with Apis.

Bites and Stings Essential Remedies

*See the chart below for specific types of bites and stings.

Apis Mel—#2 remedy for bites and stings. Redness, burning, swelling, stinging.

Arsenicum Album—bites with redness, BURNING, SWELLING, or sharp pains. May be stinging.

Belladonna—REDNESS. Sharp pains. Swelling, stinging. #1 remedy for throbbing pains.

Hypericum—sharp and shooting pains.

Arnica—#1 remedy for bites with pain.

Lachesis—Redness, swelling. Sharp pain. Stinging. BURNING.

Ledum—#1 remedy for bites and stings. Redness, burning, sharp pain, THROBBING, stinging.

Urtica Urens—redness, burning, swelling, and STINGING pains. Useful for rashes.

*Bites and Sting Remedies	General bites	Poisonous bites	Bees	Cats	Dogs	Fleas	Jellyfish	Mosquito	Rats	Scorpions	Snakes	Spiders	Wasps	Yellow jackets
Apis	X		X		X		X				X	X	X	X
Arnica	X													
Arsenicum Album	X				X						X			
Belladonna	X	X			X						X			
Hypericum	X		X	X	X	X	X		X		X	X	X	X
Lachesis	X			X	X						X			
Ledum	X	X	X	X	X	X		X	X	X		X	X	X
Urtica Urens			X				X							

BLISTERS

When the skin is irritated or burned, part of the skin layer fills with serous (clear) fluid to help repair the underlying tissue, sort of like a pillow to cushion the underlying tissue. They can be painful or painless, small or big, or in clusters. Blisters are caused by overuse or burning of skin (due to heat or sun exposure). Homeopathic remedies can help the body to heal faster and lessen the pain.

Blister Story

When people ask me about remedies for blisters, it's usually from burns. So, most of the time I will suggest Cantharis 30C—three times a day, or 200C—one or two times a day. Blisters can go away in as little as a few hours or it may take a few days. If it's been a few days since the blister formed, it will take longer. For blisters from injuries, the same healing can happen using Arnica in the same way.

Blister Essential Remedies

Antimuonium Crud—blisters from insect stings. Itching rashes. Burning. Digestive challenges.

Apis Mel—small blisters. Bee stings. Insect bites. Swelling. Stinging rash. Allergic dermatitis. Hives. BURNING, STINGING, itching, red, SWELLING.

Cantharis—sunburns. Burning and itching. RAW, SMARTING. Better from cold applications. #1 remedy for burns.

Causticum—old burns (effects from burns). Use when Antimuonium Cantharis doesn't work. Also works for incontinence.

Rhus tox—burns with small blisters. Blisters from poison ivy or poison oak. Dry, hot, burning. Red, swollen, severe itching. Burning neuralgic pains. Blisters cover abscesses. Hives. Itching better from hot water, but worse from sweating. May have arthritis.

BLOATING

Bloating is a sense of fullness and gas that builds pressure in the abdomen. It makes you feel very uncomfortable and can be accompanied by pain. Gas can put pressure on the lungs and create breathing problems; furthermore, it can put pressure on the heart causing heart-attack-like symptoms. Cause of bloating comes from eating improper foods that creates fermentation in the stomach, and small or large intestine. Included in causes are the gallbladder, liver or other reasons; other digestive organs can be weak or out of balance (stomach, pancreas, or small intestine). Antacid or PPI (proton pump inhibitor) drugs may give some temporary relief, but ultimately these cause long-term problems with mineral metabolism and are toxic. Homeopathy helps the body with digestion so that the body can relieve the symptoms.

Bloating Story
Many people suffer with bloating and abdominal discomfort. It's a common complaint these days. Western medications create a temporary relief but offer little to solve the underlying digestive issue. Carbo veg is one of the best remedies for bloating. A well-chosen remedy like this can give relief in minutes to days, and after time, as the underlying issues become solved, the remedy is no longer needed.

Bloating Essential Remedies

China/Cinchona—digestion is weak and slow, especially after eating. Heartburn with regurgitation of bitter fluid. Worse from fruit. VOMITING of undigested food. Intuitive person.

Lycopodium—bloating after eating, and from 4 to 8 P.M. Hungry at night. Eats little and feels full. Rumbling gas. Poor self-esteem. Worse from eating LEGUMES, sweets, and pastries.

Carbo Veg—#1 remedy for bloating. Slow digestion, worse one-half hour after eating. Rancid sour belching, heartburn. Lots of gas, after eating, belching, and burning. Contractive pains in the chest

---

and abdomen. Food causes sleepiness. #1 remedy for after-surgery gas pains in the shoulders.

Kali Carb—bloating after eating. Indigestion. Anxiety in stomach, gagging, bursting, sour belching. Obesity. Nausea, worse lying down. Worse from 3:00 - 4:00 A.M.

Phosphorus—bloating after eating, belching. Stomach feels hollow, cold, and empty. COLD WATER VOMITED immediately upon drinking. The sensitive person.

Causticum—bloating after eating. Salty belching. Sour belching or taste. Burning. Worse from ice water, Better from fresh meat. Often includes incontinence.

BRONCHITIS

The bronchioles are the air passageways of the upper lungs. Bronchitis is an inflammation of the bronchiole tubes. It is usually accompanied by a shallow dry cough with thick yellow mucus. The upper chest is painful. It is different from asthma, which has a wheezing or a spasmodic cough. It can also be accompanied by a common cold or a flu. Bronchitis can be a recent problem or a long-term issue. The cause is usually a cold or a virus, poor diet, inherited weakness, or lack of exercise. Homeopathics help solve underlying respiratory weakness, and symptoms are resolved in minutes or hours, with recent cases, and within a few days, gradually or sooner, in older long-lasting cases.

Bronchitis Story
Lung issues, whether it be cough, asthma, bronchitis, or pneumonia, can include the same remedies based on matching symptoms, compare them for best results. They can be used for many lung problems.

Bronchitis Essential Remedies

Most common:

Antimonium tart—bronchitis where there is RATTLING MUCUS in the upper chest. Suffocation and shortness of breath. Mucus is copious, thick and white. Croupy cough. Also use for pneumonia.

Phosphorus—bronchitis feels suffocating, hard to breathe. Whole body trembles with coughing. Person is HIGHLY SENSITIVE. Coughs up blood or rust colored mucus. Chronic bronchitis.

Other remedies:

Bryonia—bronchitis with sharp pains, difficult breathing upon any movement. MUST SIT UP TO BREATHE. Mucus looks like jelly lumps. Can't take deep breaths without coughing.

Drosera rotundifolia—bronchitis with spasmodic cough. Yellow mucus with bleeding from the nose and mouth when vomiting. Cold sweat. #1 remedy for whooping cough. Worse from talking.

Rumex crispus—bronchitis with DRY TICKLING COUGH, preventing sleep. Coughs continually, lots of mucus. Worse in cool air, at night, uncovering, drafts.

Spongia tosta—bronchitis with deep resonating dry cough. Barking CROUPY cough. Also indicated for whooping cough. Worse breathing in, before midnight, after eating, drinking, and dry cold winds.

Stannum Met—lungs feel weak, CAN HARDLY TALK. Mucus is green and has a metallic taste. Cough from laughing. Coughs easily and is hoarse.

BRUISING

Broken blood vessels cause bruising that is red, blue or black. These can be resolved in a few days or take longer to heal. Yellow coloring of a bruise is a sign it is healing. Homeopathics can help the body to rebuild tissues faster. Generally, bruising comes from mechanical injuries such as bumps and blows. Very common these days, bruising easily occurs in those taking blood thinners, which may be poorly dosed. More rarely it can be a sign of leukemia.

Bruising Story

A customer once told me about her young son who was full of energy and rarely stopped. One day he was running around the living room and fell head-first into the corner of the coffee table. Immediately, a raised bump and bruise appeared on his forehead. His mother found some Arnica homeopathic remedy and gave it to the boy. She was astonished as she watched the bruising and bump subside. Arnica Montana is the #1 remedy for bruising and soft tissue injuries. It can help healing in a few hours to days, and what's nice is that most pain goes away very quickly.

Bruising Essential Remedies

Arnica—#1 remedy for bruising. #1 remedy for soft tissue injuries. Bruises easily. Constant bruising, swelling. Injuries. Black or blue bruising. Lacerations.

Ledum—#2 remedy for bruising. Discolored, constant bruising, with swelling. Tendon injuries. BLACK EYES. Bruising from vaccinations.

Bellis Perennis—breast injury. Deep tissue injury. Soreness, swelling. Sensitive to touch. Bone bruises.

Hamamelis—constant bruising, from VARICOSE VEINS.

Phosphorus—bruise easily. Purple appearance. Bright red bruising. NOSEBLEEDS.

Ruta Grav—bruising from injuries. Itching. TENDONITIS. Mechanical injuries, often with tendonitis.

Sulphuric Acid—constant bruising. Mechanical injuries. Red, itching, blotches. Especially for internal uses (BLEEDING) such as brain hemorrhage, or other bleeding where there are fewer blood vessels, as in the eye and brain.

BURNS

Seriousness of burns ranges from skin reddening, in the first-degree, to burning pain and blistering at second-degree. Skin destruction happens at the third-degree burn. Western medicine is comparatively primitive when it comes to treating burns, and dealing with the pain and healing that requires time. I have witnessed and experienced the ability that homeopathy has to deal with burns in just a few minutes, especially when it has just happened. Burns can be caused by sun exposure, steam, scalds, chemical exposures, extreme heat, and radiation. There are remedies for all these causes. Potencies used for burns can range from 30C on up, but 200C, when used often or as needed, is best.

Burn Story

I was mowing my lawn one day and touched the engine by mistake. I heard a sizzle, then the pain came on. I rushed into the house and took Cantharis 30C and received perfect pain-symptom relief for five minutes each time I took it. Then I found a tube of Cantharis 200C and one dose took the pain and the symptoms away permanently. Several weeks later, my fingers peeled.

Burn Essential Remedies

Cantharis—#1 remedy for burns. First and second-degree burns. Prevents blistering. Chemical burns. Painful burns. Burns from steam. Scalds. Sunburn. Tongue burnt. Shock.

Calendula—use TOPICALLY, in cream or gel form; it won't allow bacteria to grow.

Belladonna—first-degree burns. Red, hot, THROBBING. Sunburn or sunstroke.

Causticum—first and second-degree burns. Burns from steam. Burns on tongue. SCALDS. Stinging burns. Chemical burns. Burns failing to heal.

Arsenicum album—first degree burns. CHEMICAL BURNS. Burning better from heat. Burns on the tongue. Scars. Old burn threatening gangrene. Restlessness. Better from warmth.

Pyrogenium—INFECTED BURNS with ulcers, abscesses, swollen, inflamed, and dry.

Phosphorus—first-degree burns. Burning. Chemical burns. Restlessness. Sensitivity. Better cold.

Kali bich—THIRD-DEGREE BURNS with yellow-green thick discharges.

CANKER SORES

Canker sores, also called "apthe," are open wounds on the inside of the mouth and on the tongue. They are painful and can burn or tingle. They may appear singly or in groups. Cankers can take up to several weeks to go away. Causation of canker sores, most of the time, is from a stomach imbalance, where the amino acid lysine is deficient. Common foods that cause canker sores include walnuts and chocolate. An anemic condition may also contribute to canker sores in the mouth. The correct homeopathic (with similar symptoms) can relieve pain in 24 hours or less and help the body heal them in as little as two days.

Canker Sores Story
I get asked frequently about painful canker sores in the mouth. A woman came to see me complaining of cankers on her tongue. Borax is

usually my first recommendation. She found the pain went away within 24 hours of using the remedy, and the sores healed up in three more days.

Canker Sore Essential Remedies

Arsenicum album—canker sores are bluish. Ulceration (break in skin). Bitter or bad taste in mouth. Cracked lips, tingling. Dry mouth. Burning. Gangrene. Pain WORSE 10 P.M. to 2 A.M. Restless perfectionist people.

Borax—cankers bleed easily. Cankers on the TONGUE and palate (roof of mouth). Cankers after eating sour and salty foods. Bitter taste in mouth. White cankers, oral thrush, fungus-like growth. Children.

Mercury Sol—cankers with EXCESSIVE SALIVA. Thirsty. Sweet or metallic taste with bad-smelling breath. Sore, red, spongy tissues. Gum boils, bleeding gums. Children and babies.

Mercury corrosive—cankers inside lips with excess saliva, and salty or metallic taste. Burning, SWOLLEN GUMS. Purple, swollen, spongy. Toothaches. Loose teeth.

Nux vomica—blood saliva at night, on pillow. Tongue and pallet slimy. White swollen gums. Sour bitter taste mornings. FOOD SITS IN THE STOMACH LIKE A ROCK. Often in children. Can also be males who crave alcohol and stimulants.

Sulphuric acid—bleeds easily, bad smelling breath. Cankers in children. On the gums, inside the lips, on the pallet. White, bloody saliva, gums bleed. Teeth rot in diabetes.

Sulphur—burning canker sores. Often in children. Inside the lips. Body feels hot. Skin problems. Gums bright red, swollen. Throbbing pains. Intellectual and unorganized person.

COLD SORES/FEVER BLISTERS

Cold sores (herpes zoster), aka fever blisters, are open wounds or crusted in the mouth, or on the lips, that are quite painful. They are associated with stress and dietary indiscretions such as too many nuts or too much chocolate. The emotional component of cold sores may represent a personal aggravation with someone close. Our lips represent our closeness to others, which is personal; we don't kiss just anyone on the lips. Cold sores are a subconscious excuse not to be close or personal. They may become worse from extra or prolonged stress.

Cold Sores Story
Solutions for cold sores are frequently requested in my store. Homeopathic Nat Mur is used with great success, especially for those who have personal, family, or love stresses. If used when the first tingle happens or is noticed, the cold sore won't even appear. If the cold sore is already apparent, it will take a day or two for symptoms such as pain to go away and a few more days for the scab to go away.

Cold Sore/Fever Blister Essential Remedies

Nat Mur—#1 remedy for cold sores/fever blisters. Most common cause is grief. INTROVERTS. Chronic cold sores from emotional issues, often caused from sun exposure, DRY LIPS, with numbness and tingling. Blisters look like pearls on lips. Round shape. Stinging pains.

Rhus tox—#2 remedy for cold sores/fever blisters. WEATHER-RELATED COLD SORES, cold damp or thunderstorms. Cold sores on the mouth and chin with dry lips. Ulcerated and corrosive, may be crusty, itching, moist, with pus coming out, burning pains. Also related to stiffness or arthritic pains.

Arsenicum album—cold sores where pains are burning, RELIEVED BY HOT APPLICATIONS. They are dry, crusty, itchy, and stinging. Perfectionism is the stress trigger.

Sepia—cold sores related to HORMONAL CHANGES. They are burning, crusty, itching, mealy, and stinging. Worse just before menstruation (hormonal change). Also introverted.

Silicea—are burning cold sores that are also corrosive, crusty, dry, itching, mealy, moist, stinging and often occur in patches. THIN, COLD, SHY people.

Sulphur—warm bodies who often have eczema. Cold sores are burning, corrosive, crusty, itching, scaly, stinging, yellow patches. Intellectual stresses are the trigger.

COLIC IN BABIES

Abdominal spasms and pains, with gas and bloating, constitute colic in babies. This can cause crying and sleeplessness. Western medicine uses PPIs (proton pump inhibitors) that disturb the true digestive power, can create kidney damage, as well as anemia and poor mineral absorption (bone health issues). Colic can come on because of a milk intolerance, or using solid foods too soon.

Colic in Babies Story
To prepare remedies for babies, take one pellet of the chosen homeopathic remedy and drop it in a 1-ounce dropper bottle filled with purified water (just to the shoulder of the bottle). Shake it until the pellet is dissolved. Give the baby a few drops in the mouth several times a day. Keep the bottle refrigerated, and make a new one each week. The right remedy will act sometimes in seconds or minutes. Be patient though, sometimes it takes more time, and acts gradually, but then resolves the colic issue for good. It works better, and safer, than a PPI (proton pump inhibitor) which only causes deeper digestive problems. You can use more than one remedy in the bottle to make your own combination.

Colic Essential Remedies

Chamomilla—#1 remedy for colic. COLIC WITH IRRITABILITY, wants to be held and reject everything. Stool looks like chopped spinach. Legs are drawn up.

Mag phos—COLIC WITH GAS. Better from bending double and heat applications. Stomach cramps. Hiccups with vomiting. Teething with spasms.

Nux vomica—irritability with colic. Weight and pain in stomach, worse morning, better eating.

Colocynthis—colic with anger. Legs are drawn up. Teething with violent pains, DOUBLES OVER, stomach cramps at night. Better from warmth.

Dioscorea*—feels better when ARCHING THE BACK (backwards). Colic with offensive gas or bad smelling gas that's sour.

Carbo veg—colic with abdominal pain, stomach cramps, gas and bloating, must bend double. Almost any FOOD CAUSES GAS and bad smelling burps. Feels sleepy after eating.

*Not in Materia Medica. Not common.

CONJUNCTIVITIS

When the conjunctiva (tissue that covers the whites of the eye) gets irritated or inflamed, you have conjunctivitis. Symptoms include redness, swelling, pain, irritation, and sometimes discharges of pus or mucus (eye can get glued shut with crusty mucus). Tears or moisture in our eyes are naturally antibacterial, but can become deficient leading to dryness. Conjunctivitis usually comes from contamination of the conjunctiva by dirty fingers. Homeopathics can quickly help the body's immune system to correct conjunctivitis in a few hours, or in a day or two. Choose the remedy that matches most closely.

Conjunctivitis

Conjunctivitis Story

Mothers are wonderful caretakers. When their children wake up with eyes glued shut, they come looking for answers. With these symptoms I will most likely suggest Pulsatilla. Pulsatilla is a great remedy that can work within a day. The child presents with symptoms of being clingy, whiny, and cries easily. Other remedies work equally well with matching symptoms.

Conjunctivitis Essential Remedies

Important: All these remedies will also have the symptom of a sand-like sensation in the eyes.

Apis mellifica—ALLERGIC PUFFY EYELIDS. Bags under eyes. Burning, stinging, hot tears. Photophobia (sensitive to strong light). Sudden piercing pains around eye sockets. Pus. CAN'T LOOK INTO ARTIFICIAL LIGHT.

Argentum nitricum—acute conjunctivitis, swelling. Discharges. Eye strain, tired eyes. Photophobia. Ulceration (open sore).

Arsenicum album—HOT BURNING EYES, better with heat. Tears irritate skin. Eyelid spasms. Stinging. Severe photophobia with sensitivity to sunlight. Yellowed discharge. Symptoms worse 10 P.M. to 2 A.M.

Pulsatilla—changeable mucus conjunctivitis with thick, bland, burning, itching. MUCUS WHICH GLUES THE EYELIDS CLOSED, upon waking in the morning. Styes. Usually weepy, whiney.

Rhus tox—eye socket cellulitis. Iritis (iris inflammation). CORNEA ULCERATION (open sore). Inflammation with blisters. Profuse tears. Paralysis in eyeball muscles. Stiff joints.

Sulphur—sand sensation in eyes. Burning, itching, quivering eyelids. Ulceration (open sore). Photophobia. Eyelids glue (gunk) up.

CONSTIPATION

If you have sluggish bowels, or are having less than one bowel movement a day, you have constipation. Some people seem pretty happy only having one bowel movement a week! There may be pain or bloating with constipation due to slow movement or a physical obstruction in the digestive system. There are many reasons why constipation is happening: it may be a poor diet, lack of fiber (or the wrong kind of fiber). Prescription medications or pain relievers, like opiates, are often involved; they slow the peristaltic movements of the bowel. Another factor could be dry bowels. Holding back, emotionally, we can become "anal-retentive." Common laxatives stimulate peristaltic movements of the bowels, but be careful as you can become dependent on them. Homeopathic remedies can help to correct the underlying causes of constipation. *See also* Bloating or Gas conditions

Constipation Story

A person came to see me wanting to stop their severe long-term constipation. The condition had started several years ago from a love loss. They became introverted and constipated. Their body and stools became dry. Nat Mur was the chosen remedy—200C potency was used just once a week. In a few weeks, regular bowel movements began happening, and the person felt emotionally much safer.

Constipation Essential Remedies

Alumina—severe obstinate constipation in INFANTS, the ELDERLY, and women who are sedentary. Severe straining to pass a soft stool. Urging precedes stool. Hard dry knotty stools. No urge to go, look like sheep dung, or covered with mucus. Severe, chronic constipation in pregnancy. Constipation from traveling.

Nat Mur—constipation from inactivity, DRYNESS, or grief. Constipation alternates days. Shyness, can't go to the bathroom around noises or other people. Constipation without urging. Worse from emotions. Worse from consolation, hates sympathy.

Nux vomica—constipation with frequent urging, but small quantities at a time; feels not enough stool has passed. Itching internal hemorrhoids. More common in MEN. Frequently uses STIMULANTS.

Sepia—Stool feels like a ball in the anus. Prolapsed rectum or anus. Oozing from anus, large hard stools. Constipation and hemorrhoids during pregnancy. Constipation with MENSTRUAL or HORMONE ISSUES. More common in females.

Silicea—constipation with constant ineffectual urging to stool. RECTAL FISSURES (deep skin cracks), painful hemorrhoids. Rectal sphincter spasms. Constipation before and during menstruation. Tendency to scarring. COLD, SHY, THIN people.

COUGHS

People cough for many reasons; it is a response due to a digestive, throat, lung, mucus or muscle spasm. Most causes of coughs are due to a respiratory problem, digestive issue (creating mucus), or muscle-related matters. Western medicine offers cough medicines that suppress the cough reflex in hopes that the body corrects itself. Side effects aren't too hazardous. However, some coughs are caused by prescription or over-the-counter drugs such as high-blood-pressure medications—so, check with your doctor. Homeopathic remedies trigger the body to correct underlying issues when you find the right remedy that matches your symptoms most closely. Some remedies work on specific types of coughs, others work on many coughs at once, as indicated below.

Cough Story
Most of my consultations about coughs are about Croupy Cough. In the 1800s, every medical doctor used Homeopathic Croup Powder consisting of Aconite, Sambucus, and Spongia Tosta. It works effectively. Results are seen usually in a day or sooner.

Cough Essential Remedies

Top three remedies that cover most coughs:

Aconite—cough caused by COLD, DRY, WINDS. Especially good for croupy cough. Most coughs. Worse lying on the back, open air, tobacco smoke, awakening from sleep, drinking cold water, and after midnight.

Drosera— Prolonged INCESSANT COUGHING. Fits of rapid coughing. Inherited lung weakness. #1 remedy for whooping cough. Most coughs. Common asthma remedy, worse from talking. Yellow mucus.

Phosphorus—cough caused by EXPOSURE TO HEAVY RAINS. Tickling coughs, worse in cold air or talking too much. Cough in the morning, or during thunderstorms. Burning dryness in the throat. Most coughs. May have a history of nosebleeds. Especially-sensitive people who are social.

Other cough remedies

Antimonium tart—Lungs feel full of mucus. Coarse, loose, RATTLING COUGH. #1 remedy for rattling cough. All kinds of lung disorders—from bronchitis or emphysema to pneumonia. Especially for infants.

Bryonia—coughs caused by taking cold drinks in hot weather. Dry HACKING PAINFUL SHARP COUGH. Worse in a warm room. Must hold chest. Pains are inside chest. Pleurisy. Everything worse by movement. Feels more on the right side of the chest.

Cuprum Met—getting wet causes coughing spasms. Cough with VIOLENT SPASMS. Out of breath. Cough gurgling sounds. Suffocative attacks at night, especially 3 A.M. Muscle cramps at night. All symptoms better cold drinks.

Hepar Sulph—coughs caused by cold dry winds. Loose cough, expectorating bloody or yellow mucus. Croupy choking cough. COUGH WHEN ANY PART OF THE BODY GETS UNCOVERED.

Ipecac—cough from overeating rich foods. Violent suffocative COUGH WITH NAUSEA AND VOMITING. Tickling, spasmodic cough, with spitting of blood. Whooping cough.

Nux vomica—cough brings on bursting headache. Dry cough at night, violent before getting out of bed. Tearing cough in chest, ripping inside chest. Mostly in males who love stimulants, alcohol.

Pulsatilla—Dry hacking coughs. Causation of cough is rich foods. CHANGEABLE SYMPTOMS. Mostly emotional women.

Rumex Crispus—DRY TICKLING COUGH, preventing sleep. Barking cough. Worse lying on left side, cool air, night, moving cold to warm rooms. Caused by uncovering, and drafts. Coughs at 11 P.M., 2 A.M., and 5 A.M. in children. Coughs continuously.

Spongia tosta—DRY, barking CROUPY cough that is worse on breathing in, and before midnight. Dry, hacking, chronic cough, may be connected to heart problems—sounds like sawing through lumber. Cough is better before eating or talking. Cough is worse in dry cold winds. #2 remedy for whooping cough. Fear of suffocating to death.

DEPRESSION

Symptoms of depression happen when someone is feeling sad. They may look sad, feel uninterested in life, isolate themselves, want to be left alone, or desire to sleep all the time. Causes of depression are many, including hormone issues, stress, abuse, loss, or physical and mental health issues. Western medicine recognizes people who have depression—they are considered "broken." They will often go through therapy and take psychotropic medicines for years or even decades. These medicines are emotionally numbing and can have sexual side-effect problems as well. Homeopathic remedies can help, even while a person is taking prescriptions for depression, as they will not interfere or interact with other medications. Using homeopathy successfully, as you find personal peace and new-found joy in life, get with your doctor to reduce medications and get on with your life!

Depression Story

A man consulted with me about his wife, who was depressed. She always felt like she had a lump in her throat and sighed often; she couldn't take a deep satisfying breath. She held resentments and felt guilty all the time. She tried Ignatia 200C, using it once a week. A few weeks passed. She reported that most of her symptoms had gone. She gave up her resentment towards her husband, and their marriage started to flourish.

Depression Essential Remedies

Aurum Met—depression not spoken about. From FINANCIAL PROBLEMS or having been let go from an important job. Also being forced to retire. FEELS SUICIDAL.

Cimicifuga—depression from disappointed love and financial concerns. It's as if a DARK CLOUD IS HANGING OVERHEAD. Feels as if they are going crazy. Pain in neck and shoulders.

Lachesis—mostly female bipolar depression. Random fast speech when stressed. Can't have anything tight around the neck. Claustrophobic. High sex drive. BIPOLAR DEPRESSION.

Lilium Tigrinum—depression from CELIBACY or lost love. Mental and physical symptoms alternate. Wants to do several things at once. Feels like they have an incurable disease. Fears going insane (also used in postpartum depression).

Nat Mur—depression from BEING HURT IN THE PAST. Can't get past their emotional sensitivity, isolates when stressed. Won't cry in public. Worse from consolation.

Nat Sulph—depression especially from a HEAD INJURY. Can have suicidal depression but doesn't go through with it because of family obligations.

Pulsatilla—depression from NOT BEING ABLE TO MAKE DECISIONS, being taken advantage of. Weepy, whiney, clinging, wants open fresh air.

Sepia—depression from HORMONAL IMBALANCES, the birth control pill, pregnancy, childbirth, or puberty. Feels like the family matters are a duty, as is sex with their partner. Wants to be alone.

Aconite—depression from a FRIGHT OR A SHOCK. Never well since fright or shock. Wants to avoid the situation.

Arsenicum album—depression from being a PERFECTIONIST. Feels restless especially from 10 P.M. to 2 A.M. Fears death or health issues for themselves and loved ones.

Ignatia—#1 remedy for acute (recent and intense) depression. The first remedy to use in acute grief. When used right away, it will help the fastest. Cries, SIGHS, has a lump in the throat.

Kali Phos—depression from stress and nervous system weakness. Used for several weeks, it will restore the nervous system.

DIAPER RASH

Symptoms of diaper rash include redness on the anus and buttocks. It can increase to blistering or bleeding, causing pain, crying, and anguish for everyone. Causes are many. It may be the mother's milk from her poor diet, or something she's eating that aggravates the baby. It could be the bottled formula that is incompatible with baby's digestive system. Also, from solid foods given too soon (less than a year after birth). Western medications used for colic, such as PPIs (proton pump inhibitors), can cause diaper rash as they disrupt healthy digestion. Teething can also cause diaper rash. Homeopathics can help baby's digestive system and diaper rash at the same time. *See also* Colic in Babies, if applicable.

Diaper Rash Story

A baby's diaper rashes are a frequent concern for new mothers. I find that Calendula Cream, applied topically, results in quick relief. Sulphur is most commonly used as the first remedy. Other remedies may be indicated, by their symptoms, for a more permanent effect. Important: Babies can't tell us their symptoms. Take cues from when they cry out, as it may be an ulceration (open wound) which is painful. More than rashes do, cutting pains will hurt more when the child moves.

Diaper Rash Essential Remedies

Use Calendula Cream, topically, along with these diaper rash remedies:

Graphites—rectal fissures (deep skin cracks) bleed. Large, difficult, bad-smelling stools. Diaper RASH CAUSES PUS; moist, crusty eruptions, and a sticky ooze.

Sulphuric Acid—sour smell. Oozing, bruising, red skin. Can have boils. Itching blotches.

Mercury Sol—skin moist, itching worse from warmth of the bed. Ulceration (break in skin), bleeding, cutting pains, PROUD FLESH. Rawness and burning. Green slimy stools.

Mercury Corrosive—blisters, ULCERATIONS (breaks in skin), itching, eruptions, boils. Better with coldness. Excessive irritating sweat, causing pain. All symptoms worse from sweating.

Muriatic Acid—smarting and burning pains, small blisters, itching.

Nitricum Acid—SPLINTER-LIKE SHARP PAINS with bleeding. Rash has distinct edges, itching. Anal fissures (deep skin cracks).

Sulphur—use this remedy if nothing else works, or, in addition to other remedies. Red hot skin, red itching anus. Dry scaly skin. Worse from heat.

DIARRHEA

Poorly formed stools, liquid stools, explosive or undigested-food stools, as well as mucous in stools, all constitute diarrhea. There may be pain, or no pain at all. Feeling weak after diarrhea is possible. Diarrhea has many causes. Mostly, it's caused by digestive issues involving the stomach, liver, gallbladder, small intestines, or large intestine. There can be irritation of any of these organs. Medications may be a cause, especially antibiotics. Colds, flu, bacterial infection or other infections may be a cause too. Food poisoning is often a cause. You may never know the real cause. In homeopathy, we look to match the symptoms the person is having to choose the best remedy, and the body will take care of the rest.

Diarrhea Story

The most common homeopathic for diarrhea is Podophyllum 30C, taken at two pellets three times a day for two to three days. If it is not working, look for a better symptom match in another remedy. Results can be very good. Beware of diarrhea in small children. Check with your doctor if symptoms don't improve in a day or two.

Diarrhea Essential Remedies

Arsenicum Album—diarrhea from FOOD POISONING. Burning, thin, rice-water stools, with bloody mucus. Exhaustion. Nausea or vomiting. Food poisoning. Perfectionist, anxious. Worse 10 P.M. to 2 A.M.

Nat Sulph—diarrhea, especially on waking or after breakfast. With gas. Stool loose with bloody mucus. Worse in damp weather or in summer drinking cold drinks. Also used for head injuries, depression.

Phosphorus—painless diarrhea that is EXHAUSTING. Diarrhea that is uncontrollable; rectum-open sensation. Stool bloody, or lumps of mucus. Sensitive people who are intuitive and social, they may take on other people's emotional baggage.

Podophyllum—#1 remedy for diarrhea. First remedy to try. Diarrhea with IBS (irritable bowel), colitis, diverticulitis. Lots of gas, sputtering, messy, and loud. Happens at 4 to 5 A.M. or 4 to 5 P.M. Can't tell if they want to vomit or pass a stool. Exhausting. Yellow, bad-smelling stool.

Sulphur—involved with bowel diseases, worse from heat, beer. Waking with diarrhea at 6 A.M. Smells like rotten eggs or Sulphur. Bleeding in stool, or mucus. Intellectual, social people, confused by too many ideas.

Veratrum Album—history of bowel problems. Vomiting and diarrhea at the same time. Diarrhea is bloody, black, and acidic. No odor. Very religious people.

EARACHES (EAR INFECTIONS)

Earaches can happen in either ear, or both. Ear canals or eardrums may be filled with mucus. Sometimes, earaches can lead to deafness if left unchecked. There is a tenderness when touching the bone behind the ear, or pain while tugging on the earlobe, or outside of the Eustachian tube. The eardrum can be red and swollen. Earaches can be caused by infection in the ear canal or behind the eardrum, from improper diet or some other bacterial or viral infection. The cause of these infections is not always known, but can be improved by eating a better diet. The correct homeopathic remedy can relieve symptoms, sometimes in minutes or hours. Hot packs on the affected ear can give temporary relief. You can still give homeopathic remedies with antibiotics if necessary—they will not interfere or interact and often give extra help. Give homeopathic remedies in a 6C or 30C potency every couple of hours.

Earache Story

Earaches are a big topic of concern for parents dealing with young children. Right-sided earache with fever, and the right cheek being red, frequently responds quickly when using Belladonna. A Chamomilla earache will usually be accompanied by irritating diarrhea that looks like spinach. The child wants to be held, but is very irritable. You'll see relief in minutes when the right remedy is given.

Earache Essential Remedies—recent intense or long lasting

Acute (recent intense) Earache Remedies

Belladonna—RIGHT-SIDED earache, right cheek red, with THROBBING PAIN. Ears hot and sensitive, cries out in sleep due to delirium. Worse with noises, being bumped, heat. Also, worse 3 to 11 P.M. and during the night.

Chamomilla—VERY IRRITABLE, but wants to be held. With fever and pain, sensitive. Worse with music. Green stools.

Pulsatilla—wants to be held and loved. External ears are swollen and red. Ear infections worse at night. Not better from hot applications.

Hepar Sulph—ear painful, sensitive to touch, and from DRAFTS. Very irritable with much anger.

Mercury Sol—EARDRUM RUPTURES with yellow pus or bloody discharges. Eustachian tubes blocked and painful in warmth of bed or heat. Sharp or shooting pains. Everything is worse at night. Also for chronic ear infections.

Chronic (long-lasting) Earache Remedies

Mercury Sol—same as acute.

Kali Sulph—Eustachian tube deafness. Bad-smelling discharges—yellow, watery, sticky, thin.

Silicea—PERFORATED EARDRUMS. Puts fingers in ears. Ear discharges smell bad. Hissing or roaring in the ears. Weak, thin, cold, shy person who is sick all the time.

Chamomilla—same as acute.

Pulsatilla—same as acute.

ECZEMA

In eczema, the skin can be dry, red, bordered, blistered, crusty, or have eruptions. Eczema can be acute, which means it comes intensely and leaves quickly, or can come on slowly and stay for a long time, which is chronic. It can cause itching or even pain. Causes are often bad diets (nutrition failure) and a general breakdown of the skin, superficial or deep. Eczema can be caused by the body's inability to detoxify itself—the liver may have a weakness and must be helped. Western medications are prescribed in topical application (on the skin). These topical medications contain steroids that only temporarily help the symptoms and may cause toxicity or lung damage. Then asthma appears, where a person will need to use steroid inhalers [not a good idea in my mind]. Homeopathic remedies may help break the cycle of steroid use and help the body to recover. Use homeopathic remedies in low potency of 6C or 30C once or twice a day. The results might either be gradual or rather quick. Gradual results are the norm. If you have an aggravation where symptoms become worse, don't worry. It is the body pushing toxins to the surface to get rid of them. Normally, something like this will last a day or two, then the eczema will improve. If it doesn't, stop the remedy and try another. For eczema, in general, stay away from creams, salves, and especially steroid applications.

Eczema Story

I have encountered several eczema cases where Petroleum was the remedy that helped. The main symptom is deep cracks on the tops of the hands and fingers. When the hands are clenched, these cracks break open and bleed, and it is quite painful. The eczema is always worse in winter. My favorite story is about a five-year-old boy who had eczema over his entire body. He had the typical symptoms in his hands, whereby any time he moved or bent his fingers, he was opening cracks, breaking scabs and bleeding. And yes, crying out in pain every time. He had had copious amounts of steroid creams used on his skin. His doctor determined the boy was too toxic, so his mother gave up using the creams. She gave him Petroleum 30C twice a day for a month. When he came back in with her, he could clinch his hands without them cracking open, and half of his eczema was gone! He jumped around the office like a normal five-year-old boy. It was exciting to see.

Eczema Essential Remedies

Sulphur—the FIRST REMEDY used for eczema: 6C two times a day for a couple of weeks, or use in conjunction with other remedies. Unhealthy skin. Every injury opens up. Itching, burning. Worse from warmth. Intellectual, but untidy person.

Arsenicum Album—eczema alternates with asthma. Skin itching, burning, swelling, dry, rough, scaly, worse from cold. Better from heat. Anxious especially after 10 P.M. Hives from shellfish. PERFECTIONIST.

Calc Carb—damp cold hands, weak ankles. Stinging rash, better from cold air. Boils, Petechia- red spots, raised. The homebody with TENDENCY TO OBESITY.

Graphites—ECZEMA IN FOLDS OF SKIN. Obesity with eczema. Thickened, dry, rough skin. Every wound will pus, get crusty, and weep or ooze yellow honey-like discharge, especially behind the ears. Cracks in skin. Old scars open. Worse from heat. Moody.

Hepar Sulph—every wound produces pus, boils, abscess, ulcers. Hives. Deep cracks. Wants to be wrapped up warmly. EASILY IRRITABLE. Worse from cold dry wind.

Mezereum—Oozing, irritating, gluey discharges that create a THICK YELLOW CRUST with pus underneath. Intolerable itching, worse from warmth of bed. Skin can break down to resemble fish scales. Hypochondriac (worries about health unnecessarily). Irritable.

Petroleum—eczema with CRACKS IN SKIN, bleeds easily. Worse cold damp weather (WINTER). Parchment skin. Skin won't heal. Thick greenish crust, burning, itching, bleeding, red, even clothes rubbing is irritating.

Rhus tox—eczema worse from WEATHER CHANGES, cold, and damp. Eczema red, swollen, itching, burning. Nerve pains. May also have arthritic stiffness of joints. Poison ivy-like hives. Itching better in hot water. Scale formation.

EXHAUSTION

Feeling so fatigued that you are not able to perform daily tasks, or can't think clearly, or don't have enough energy to get up and do something—all these symptoms point to exhaustion. There are many reasons for exhaustion. For some people it is unnecessarily overworking for weeks and sometimes years; night watching or insomnia, loss of sleep in general; caretaking; allergies or hay fever from pollen; chemicals; food sensitivities; emotions such as grief; medications; adrenal exhaustion. Low iron or anemia can also be a factor. There must be many questions asked of the person who is exhausted. We can match key symptoms and find solutions with homeopathy.

Exhaustion Story

I consult, a great deal, with people who are exhausted. I ask a lot of questions. A woman, who came in with her husband, complained that he didn't have the "energy" to satisfy her intimately. He worked 12-hour days doing cement work. He and I talked. He agreed to cut back to working 8 hours per day, and began to use Arnica 30C, 3 times a day. After a few days, he began to have enough "energy" for his wife.

Exhaustion Essential Remedies

Acute (recent)

Arnica—exhaustion from over-exercising or injury. Bruised sensation. Bruising. Bed feels too hard. PHYSICAL OVERWORKED.

Kali Phos—exhaustion from weakness of the nervous system, stress, excitement, or mentally overworked. Easily fatigued.

Picric Acid—exhausted from test fears, memory weakness, BRAIN FATIGUE. Too much mental work.

Gelsemium—exhaustion from PANIC ATTACKS, fright, fear, bad news. Internal shaking from thinking of future stressful events such as public speaking or going to the dentist.

Arsenicum album—exhaustion from anxiety and fear of death. The PERFECTIONIST. Doing too much, too many hours worked, too many projects. Anxiety worse 10 P.M. to 2 A.M.

China/Cinchona—exhaustion from LOSS OF FLUIDS (liquid or blood loss, dehydration), also food poisoning. Sweating excessively can cause weakness.

Phosphoric Acid—exhaustion when MENTAL OVERWORKING causes depression, or depression causes exhaustion, or mental overwork causes physical exhaustion.

Silicea—exhaustion in weak, THIN, SHY people who have skin problems.

FEVERS

Fever is a rise in body temperature with discomfort, possible sweating, and exhaustion. Fevers are a natural body defense. When the body temperature rises, the immune system is more effective and pathogens such as bacteria or viruses are less effective. So, homeopathic remedies work in fevers because they help the immune system, and then the fever is no longer needed.

Fever Story

The social group that experiences fevers the most are children. Homeopathic remedies help the body's immune system to reduce the fever effectively in just a few hours. A great fever combination is low, medium, and high-fever cell salts (6X potency) or homeopathic remedies which include Ferrum Phos, Kali Mur, and Kali Sulph. Take all together every 2 or 3 hours.

Fever Essential Remedies

Top Fever Remedies

Aconite—low fever of 99-101 degrees Fahrenheit. High anxiety with fever. Dry fever, worse evenings. Fever from exposure to cold dry winds.

Gelsemium—low fever of 99-102 degrees Fahrenheit. Fever with a cold or flu. Shakiness inside. Exhaustion. Apathetic, dull, with fever and chills. High fevers worse at night.

Other Fever Remedies

Belladonna—sudden-onset high fever of 103-106 degrees Fahrenheit. Right cheek is hot, the other is cool. PAIN IS THROBBING, which is a sign of inflammation, with sweating. Severe throbbing headaches worse at night with chills. Worst nights and afternoons.

Ferrum Phos (also a cell salt)—sudden low fever of 99-101 degrees Fahrenheit. Or, slow-onset fever. First stage of a cold or flu or inflammation. Paleness alternating with redness.

Kali Mur (also a cell salt)—medium fever of 101-103 degrees Fahrenheit. Second stage of cold or flu, usually taken with Ferrum Phos. Used for fevers with white mucus and respiratory issues.

Kali Sulph (also a cell salt)—high fever of 103-105 degrees Fahrenheit. Yellow mucus discharges with high fever. Rattling mucus in chest, sore throat (Ant Tart). Wandering pains (Pulsatilla).

FLU

Viral flu symptoms can be achiness, fever, loss of smell or taste, mucus of several kinds, and loss of respiratory function. Symptoms also may include nasal congestion and swollen glands. There are often chills, exhaustion, muscle aches. There are over 300 types of flu viruses that affect humans. They are all spread by personal contact and water droplets.

Flu

Poor immune health and nutritional deficiencies may also contribute. Stress and sleep deprivation contribute to vulnerability and susceptibility to viruses as well.

Flu Story
Homeopathics are often used to help the immune system deal with viruses more efficiently and cut short the symptoms. When you can find the similar homeopathic remedy, the symptoms can go away within a couple of days. A few years ago, I found a homeopathic remedy that worked for almost everyone (sometimes a single remedy will fit the symptoms of that year's flu outbreak), where symptoms went away in 24 to 48 hours. Find the remedy that best matches your symptoms. It doesn't hurt to try any of the remedies listed below.

Flu Essential Remedies

Arsenicum album—Stomach flu with diarrhea and BURNING PAINS, nausea. Much thirst for sips of warm drinks. Anxious and restless. Chills and fever with diarrhea. All symptoms are worse at night, and from 10 P.M. to 2 A.M. Also good for food poisoning.

Baptisia*—sudden onset, deeper, more severe flu (when Gelsemium is not strong enough, but may follow Gelsemium to finish the flu off). High fever and great weakness. Feels and looks drunk, confused, delirious, inability to think. Thirst for small amounts. CAN SWALLOW LIQUIDS ONLY, as solid food gags. TOXIC APPEARANCE—body odor, breath, stool, all bad smelling. Food poisoning or bad water. Septic conditions, great muscle soreness. Worse on awakening, with cold wind, thinking of pain, humidity, indoors, and pressure.

Bryonia—Slow onset flu. Splitting headache worse from any motion. All pains and symptoms are sharp and WORSE WITH ANY MOVEMENT; deep breathing hurts. Chill with external coldness and internal heat. Limbs and joints ache. Severe dryness of lips, throat and mucus membranes. Thirsty, craves cold drinks. Dry hacking cough—holds chest when coughing. Better from pressure. Irritable and frustrated. Constipation with dry hard stools.

Eupatorium Perf—high fevers. Fever and chills alternate. Sick and sweaty. Thirsty for cold drinks. Throbbing bursting headaches. BONES ACHE as if they would break; deep in the bones, back and legs. Chills preceded by thirst and aching soreness of bones. Worse from cold air and motion. Symptoms occur periodically. Worse in the morning, chills between 7 and 9 A.M.

Gelsemium—slow onset flu with no fever and dry cough, sore chest and mucus discharge from stuffy nose. TREMBLING AND SHAKING, muscle aches and weakness. No thirst. Dizzy, droopy feeling. Drowsy with eyelids half-closed. Blurry vision. Flu associated with nervous stress, fear, fright, emotional excitement or upset. Very apathetic. Wiped-out feeling, dullness, can't exert self or move. Chills run up and down the spine as if cold water were poured down the back.

Phosphorus—very weak; empty, gone sensation felt in stomach. Cold fluid is thrown up as soon as it gets in a warm stomach. Talking painful. TIGHTNESS ACROSS CHEST, great weight on chest. Hard, dry, tight racking cough. Congestion of the lungs. Craves cold ice drinks. body trembles with a cough. Can hardly hold anything with hands as arms and hands become numb. Exhaustion from diarrhea. Burning heat up back.

Rhus Tox—slow onset flu, especially from physical overexertion in the cold damp. Swollen glands, sore sticking pains with swallowing. Hoarseness with loss of voice. Chilly as if cold water poured over them, followed by heat. Restlessness, has to keep moving. Tongue coated with a red tip, dry edges. Vertigo on rising. Tickling sensation behind the sternum (chest). Aching and stiffness of limbs, sore joints, wants to stretch—worse on first motion but better by continued motion. Aching in all bones (Eupatorium). WORSE COLD DAMP WEATHER.

*Not in Materia Medica. Not common.

GALLSTONES

Gallstones start first with indigestion, and can cause a bitter taste in the mouth. There can be sharp pain under the lower right ribs and tenderness of the tip of the right shoulder blade. Pain can be unbearable, worse with eating fatty foods. The cause of gallstones is often a poor diet (including fried foods), too many beans or legumes, and excess amounts of coffee. The liver may be impaired and not producing enough bile to keep the body from producing gallstones. Adequate bile flow prevents sludge and gallstone build-up. Bile is used to break down fats, and is transportation for toxin breakdown from the liver. It is also lubricant for the intestines to help with normal bowel movements. Western medicine often removes the gallbladder. Research indicates gallbladder removal will help a person feel better one-third of the time, not feel better one-third of the time, and actually feel worse one-third of the time. *See also* Bloating and Gas conditions.

Gallstone Story

I receive frequent phone calls for gallstone problems, especially when people are in pain. The most frequent complaints are pain and tenderness on the bottom tip of the right shoulder blade. I have suggested the remedy Chelidonium frequently, with good results. Most people feel better in a few days. Then they use it for another month and the symptoms usually don't return. Other remedies may be indicated. These homeopathics stimulate the liver to produce a healthy amount of bile so the gallbladder functions normally.

Gallstone Essential Remedies

Berberis vulgaris—used for any kind of stones, often used for the left kidney, with RADIATING PAIN, sciatica and nerve problems. Symptoms worse with pressure, motion; pain prevents normal breathing. Clay-colored stools and jaundice or yellow skin.

Calc Carb—symptoms with obesity, and weak ankles. SYMPTOMS FROM OVERWORK. Skin smells sour. Feels weak, tired. Worse in cold, motion, pressure of clothes. Lots of health fears. Colocynthis—Lower abdominal cramping. Feels better from hot packs or wrapped in general. Worse from emotions such as anger, frustration. Pain, doubles over.

Lycopodium—symptoms worse from 4 to 8 P.M. with indigestion. Right-sided pains, worse lying on the right side.

Nat Sulph—has liver and gallbladder problems. Symptoms worse 4 to 5 A.M. Can be associated with head injuries. Symptoms worse dampness and cold.

China/Cinchona—NEVER WELL SINCE GALLBLADDER SURGERY. Has gas but doesn't feel better passing gas. Feels bloated. Hypersensitive to touch, must loosen clothing. Deep pressure feels better. Feels better with fasting.

GAS

Gas and bloating can cause the upper or lower abdomen to distend or expand. It may produce an uncomfortable feeling and is often relieved by passing gas. Gas can also get trapped and cause pain. Gas passed can be silent or noisy, odorless or bad smelling. No one is happy. Causes of gas and bloating are poor diet, poor digestion—or both. Certain foods can cause gas such as beans, etc. Low stomach acid may also be a factor; it can cause fermentation of food not being broken down, and which causes gas. Prescriptions or over-the-counter medications, such as antacids or PPI (proton pump inhibitors) medications, can worsen digestion. Episodes of gas and bloating can last from a few minutes to weeks, and even months. The situation can be so bad that the stomach can expand and put pressure on the lungs making breathing harder, or put pressure on the heart, even causing heart-attack-like symptoms. *See also* Gas or Colic in Babies conditions.

Gas Story
Some time ago a man complained to me that he shared an office with his brother, who he threatened to kick him out, as his brother was passing "silent, but deadly" (he called it) gas. I suggested Nux Vomica 30C, three times a day, and, it worked in less than a day. He was forever grateful.

Gas Essential Remedies

Argentum Nit—anticipation gas is loud but gives relief, usually without odor. Over sensitive to sweets. Anxious with a tendency to panic attacks. Craves sweets.

Carbo Veg—hot moist offensive gas. Passing gas gives relief. Irritating, BURNING FLUIDS FROM RECTUM WHEN PASSING GAS. Stools smell like death.

Colocynthis—gas worse from anger. Musty odor. Constipation with hard stools. Bad OFFENSIVE SMELL.

Lycopodium—low self-esteem, gas worse from legumes. Right-side (liver issues). Bad offensive smell. Worse 4 to 8 P.M.

Nat Sulph—gas from liver issues. Head injuries. Very bad-smelling gas. BETTER FROM PASSING GAS.

Nux-vomica—gas from stimulants, alcohol. Liver impairment with bad gas. FOOD SITS IN THE STOMACH LIKE A ROCK. Mostly males.

Phosphorus—feels better when passing gas. Sensitive to emotions, picks up on other people's problems.

GOUT

Symptoms of gout include sharp, excruciating pains in the joints. There may be swelling and redness. Every pain is worse upon movement. Classic gout is debilitating pain in the big toes that's worse with the least touch or motion. Western medicines for gout are generally toxic, and rarely get to the root cause. Homeopathy, however, can help the body in just a few days, by relieving the symptoms of pain. Gout causes in the body are from a combination of eating foods rich in uric acid, and the kidneys inability to release uric acid into the urine and into the toilet. Foods rich in uric acid include pork, beef, and sardines, among others. You may need to forgo these foods to allow the kidneys to recover and pass uric acid normally.

Gout Story

Some cultural groups have a tendency to gout. I have been consulted by many people from this group. I have often seen Colchicum 30C, taken two to three times a day, give relief in hours to days. If that does not give relief for you, other remedies can be effective upon closer symptom match.

Gout Essential Remedies

Colchicum—#1 remedy for gout. Screams in pain, when touching affected part, worse at night. Typically, pains of PINS AND NEEDLES IN THE BIG TOES. Kidney failure with pain. Nausea at night, or from the smell of food.

Arnica—gout especially from injuries or overexertion. BRUISED FEELING. Joint and muscle pain. Loss of strength.

Benzoic Acid—gout in kidney weakness, URINE SMELLS STRONG. Bedwetting. Joints crack, especially in the elderly. Pains in Achilles tendon. Bunions. Ganglion cysts. Tearing pain.

Bryonia—gout when motion makes symptoms sharp and painful. Involuntary urination. Joints red, swollen. Hot swelling of feet.

Lycopodium—gout when there is liver involvement and symptoms worse from 4 to 8 P.M. Sciatica right side. Heel pain. Low self-esteem.

Nux Vomica—gout with liver involvement, caused by stimulants, especially ALCOHOL ABUSE. Unable to urinate, leg cramps, knee joints crack.

Rhus Tox—gout with STIFFNESS, cracking of joints. Worse from storms and cold damp conditions.

GRIEF

Grief and sadness can show symptoms including: crying, loss of emotion, insomnia, memory loss, loss of sex drive, loss of joy in general. It can be exhausting. Grieving can take weeks, to months, to years, or never finish. From a Western medical perspective, many people are prescribed antidepressants, anti-anxiety drugs, or worse. And, at best, a person feels numbed inside. Even worse, these medications don't clear the grief, and also bring severe side effects. They prolong the grieving process. Everyone on this planet will experience a traumatic event in life, such as losing a loved one, friend, colleague, or even a beloved animal. The body will go into a defense mode and experience the above symptoms of grief. Homeopathy is a wonderful tool for grief and has been used for a couple of hundred years to help the person (body and spirit) deal with dramatic emotion without suppressing grief or having side effects.

Grief Story
I have suggested the remedy Ignatia many times. When used soon after love loss or death of a loved one, there is more sweetness in the

memories than the normal bitterness. It generally works in minutes to hours. To see my clients or friends find relief from this acute grief is immensely satisfying.

Grief Essential Remedies

Aurum Met—worried about FINANCIAL LOSS causes grief and depression. #1 remedy for suicidal depression. Won't talk about problems. Grief in BUSINESS PEOPLE, from a loss. From divorces, grief about the future, loses sleep.

Ignatia—#1 remedy for acute grief following DEATH OF A LOVED ONE. Sighing, crying, lump in throat, hard to take a deep breath. Mental breakdown. Also, silent grief, death, divorce, hurt feelings, and from past hurts with sleeplessness.

Nat Mur—mostly CHRONIC GRIEF, silent grief with sleeplessness, weakness. Relieves grief from old love losses or emotional traumas by crying alone (not in public). Emotionally sensitive. Isolates when stressed. Physical manifestations are cold sores (fever blisters), and cravings for salt and salty foods. Dryness or clear nasal mucus discharges. Hates consolation.

Phosphoric acid—grief and depression from too much MENTAL WORK and oversensitivity. From love loss, homesickness—becomes apathetic or indifferent. Weak feeling in chest when talking.

Pulsatilla—grief can cause diarrhea, weight loss, SILENT SUFFERING—from a divorce, silent grieving. Talks about deceased. Crying, whiny, doesn't want to be alone, people pleaser. Wants attention and consolation. Symptoms are changeable.

Staphysagria—grief from being a victim of EMOTIONAL OR SEXUAL ABUSE, or is presently in an abusive situation. Has been humiliated. Grief from a divorce. Feels emotional pain, especially old emotional hurts.

GUMS

What happens in our mouths is related to our overall health. Science has revealed that gum health and heart health are connected. Gum symptoms can include inflammation and soreness, bleeding easily; can be spongy, ooze pus, turn a variety of colors, and also be painful. They can also decay or recede and expose teeth roots. If you brush your teeth too hard you may cause the gums to recede. If you don't floss regularly the gums may be tender and bleed easily. Certain underlying nutritional and health conditions may contribute to your gum health and can jeopardize your teeth, which can become loose and may fall out. I have seen homeopathy help gums if the remedies are well-chosen. *See also* Toothaches, if applicable.

Gum Story
One of my clients asked about receding gums after visiting her dentist. I recommended Mercury Sol 30C, two pellets two times a day. After three months she returned to her dentist. He was impressed and requested to use it for his own gum health. The client said her gums improved and no longer bled.

Gum Essential Remedies

Calc Carb—bleeding gums with SOUR taste and smell. Tongue dry at night, tip of tongue burning. Workaholic. Family oriented. Obesity.

Carbo veg—cold, bad breath with bitter and sour taste in mouth. Loose teeth from spongy gums that bleed. Gums retracted and black. Gum boils bluish-black cankers. GAS, bloating. Apathy, anxiety mornings.

Kali Phos—gums are receding, spongy, with red line on gum. Cankers, bad breath. DRY, especially mornings. nervous exhaustion from overwork.

Kreosotum—bitter taste, gums are puffy, oozing, spongy, bleeding, and affect the teeth with rapid decay. Gums puffy and bluish. Obstinate, denies bad health. Systemic breakdown.

Lachesis—gums swollen, PURPLE, spongy, bleeding. Crumbling teeth, bad breath. Sour, metallic burning taste. Left-sided. Talkative. Can't stand anything around the neck.

Mercury Sol— cankers, painful gums, spongy and receding gums, gum boils. SWEET and metallic taste. Loose teeth. Gums swell at night. Excess saliva. Bad breath. Restless, changeable, poor self-confidence.

Mercury Corr—gums purple, spongy, swollen. Salty saliva (Nat Mur). Metallic taste. Bitter. Burning mouth. Loose teeth. Cankers. Restless, irritable, bad digestion.

Nat Mur—gums spongy, bleeding, gum boils. Bad breath. LOSS OF TASTE AND SMELL. DRY SKIN, or EXCESS BODILY FLUIDS (runny nose, watery eyes, lots of saliva). Cankers. Introvert, sensitive, won't show feelings. Depression.

Nitric Acid—bloody saliva, especially inner gums, swollen, sore. Bad breath. Yellow teeth, loose. SPLINTER PAINS. Gums white, itching and bleeding. NEGATIVE pessimistic attitude.

Phosphorus—gums bleed, swollen, ulcerated. Gum boils. Excessive salty saliva. Rotten-egg taste mornings. Sour taste after milk. Cankers. SENSITIVE, poor boundaries, hard to make decisions.

Silicea—gum boils, sensitive to air and cold water. Excessive saliva, dry mouth. Gangrene ulcers. THIN, COLD, SHY PEOPLE.

Sulphur—HOT, copious saliva, bleeding gums, throbbing pains. Gum boils. Intellectual and untidy people.

HAY FEVER/ALLERGIES

Hay fever symptoms first include low energy, and the memory and thinking are affected. Next symptoms are the sneezing, coughing, mucus, red eyes, and itching. Causes of hay fever may be food sensitivities, pollens, chemicals, dust, or wind. These causes trigger the mast cells (trillions of them from the nose to the gastrointestinal tract, to the anus). When affected, they degranulate and release histamines that cause inflammation and common hay fever symptoms. Western medicine uses antihistamines that block the inflammatory response, but may cause cognitive decline and other toxicities in the body. Homeopathic remedies help relieve symptoms and the underlying sensitivities, along with effecting better mast cell stability.

Hay Fever Story

The most common hay fever complaint is itching, burning eyes. Allium cepa fits this symptom and gives relief. A 30C potency, two pellets three times a day—or as needed—helps relieve symptoms in minutes to hours. It is not generally for the underlying causes; for that you need a remedy that matches the symptoms more closely.

Hay Fever Essential Remedies

Allium cepa—allergic constitution. Eyes sensitive, BURNING TEARS. Lots of bland tears. Hoarseness. Fall or spring allergies, nose drips, sneezing in a warm room, with discharges burning and irritating the nose and upper lip. Sinusitis. Asthma.

Arsenicum album—thin watery excoriating. Hoarseness. Burning. Itching. Sneezing without relief. Asthmatic. Worse in springtime. The perfectionist. Anxious especially 10 P.M. to 2 A.M.

Sabadilla—FREQUENT SPASMODIC SNEEZING. Runny nose. Copious watery discharge. Over sensitivity to odors. Dry itching and tickling of nose. Asthmatic in springtime. Worse from odor of flowers or thinking of them.

Arsenicum Iod—swollen nose. Burning irritating tears. Desire to sneeze. Chronic nasal mucus. Nasal ulcers. Wheezing when first lying down. Chronic asthma. Chronic hay fever.

Nat Mur—watery discharges from eyes and nose. VIOLENT SNEEZING. Sinusitis. Loss of smell and taste. Chronic hay fever. Craves salt. Introvert. Sensitive, but won't cry in public.

Nat Sulph—hay fever from liver issues. Congested nose and sinus. Dryness. Burning. Discharges thick yellow and salty. Sneezing. Asthmatic. Watery discharges night, or during menstruation. Symptoms randomly stop and start.

HEAD INJURIES

Head injuries, also referred to as TBI (traumatic brain injury) can have a wide range of symptoms. First is pain, then disorientation, then unconsciousness (temporary). Those with head injuries may recover; some may never recover. Long-term problems may include: memory loss or weak memory, with specific areas of thinking affected; vertigo, loss of balance, depression and suicidal thoughts. Some people experience vision disturbances or vision loss. Emotional change can also be seen. One may also be unable to keep their employment, or even relationships. Trauma to the head can happen with, or without, going unconscious. Western medicine is important for emergency purposes. Help for longer-standing brain injuries may come in the form of antidepressant drugs, but they always carry side effects and toxicity. Homeopathy can help the victim of TBIs in amazing ways. It is best used right after the injury, but can be helpful even years later.

Head Injury Story
Among the countless success stories on head injuries, Nat Sulph stands out the most. A woman called me two weeks after she was in a car accident. She suffered a concussion. She had also lost most of her sight, and the diagnosis from doctors was not encouraging. At my suggestion

she used Nat Sulph 200C, at one-week intervals. The next week, she announced to me that her vision was back to normal. She then complained that her memory was still a bit foggy. That, too, mostly cleared up in another three weeks.

Head Injury Essential Remedies (also injury from head surgery)

Arnica—ailments after concussion. Epilepsy. #1 remedy for head injury: start with Arnica. Loss of voice, hoarseness. Headaches, dullness, memory loss. Depression. Deafness. Vertigo. Pain after injury.

Cicuta—ailments after concussion. EPILEPSY. Pain after injury. Vertigo after. Arches spine. CONVULSIONS. Catalepsy (sits staring). Screaming. Headache. Depression. Memory problems. Stuttering.

Helleborus—ailments after concussion, epilepsy. STUTTERING. Mental symptoms, memory loss. STUPEFIED, dull, slow to answer. Apathetic. Automatic chewing. Brain cry, frowning. alteration of consciousness.

Hypericum—ailments after concussion. Epilepsy, seizures. Pain after. Mental issues, depression, dullness, memory loss. Depression. HEAD AND SPINAL INJURIES. Rigid. Nerve pains. Nerve damage.

Nat Sulph—#1 remedy for head injuries, and after-effects of head injuries. Ailments after concussion, epilepsy. Mental symptoms, memory loss. Pains after, vertigo after. Blindness. Coma. Depression, suicidal depression. Petit Mal absence seizures. Sensitivity to music. Worse damp weather, headaches, dullness.

Sulphuric acid—CLEARS INTRACRANIAL (IN-BRAIN) BLEEDING. Brain damage symptoms, changes in personality. Confused, disoriented, slurred speech, hearing problems, impaired balance, impaired breathing with irregular pauses. Heart rhythm disturbances.

HEADACHES

People have many different types of headaches with symptoms consisting of all kinds of pains, in different bodily locations, at different times of day, and of different sensitivities. There are regular headaches, migraine headaches, headaches with possible vision or other secondary problems—a diverse sample. Western medicine uses pain relievers, caffeine, and other drugs that temporarily relieve symptoms. Causes of headache are as diverse as the symptoms; it could be a result of chemical sensitivities, digestion, menstrual or hormonal issues, and many others. Fortunately, homeopathy can help the body to address underlying issues by matching remedies with symptoms. Results, or relief, can be quick or gradual. The remedies listed here are the most common. For best results seek a homeopath.

Headache Story

A woman came to see me who was a healthcare worker. She was desperate for help, but somewhat hostile to the "alternative medicine" of homeopathy. She had a 24/7 migraine for 20 years, from the time she was 6. Western medicine had no answers for her. In our fifteen-minute consultation, she described her one-sided migraine that throbbed to the beat of her heart. Clearly that fit the symptoms of the remedy Glonoinum. I had some of this remedy, so she wanted to try it right then. And, as we continued to speak, the pain went away in less than ten minutes. She then continued using Glonoinum 30C, two pellets three times a day, and in only one month the headache went away permanently.

Headache Essential Remedies (Migraines included)

Belladonna—RIGHT-SIDED THROBBING headaches. Right cheek red, hot. Worse from motion. Congestive headaches especially in the forehead. Pain worse with light and noise, jarring, lying down, afternoon, haircuts, draft, or washing hair. Sudden onset.

Bryonia—SHARP PAINS WORSE BY MOVEMENT. More right-sided. Migraines, bursting, splitting, frontal headaches, scalp sensitive. Vertigo, nausea.

Glonoinum—right-sided, THROBS TO THE BEAT OF THE HEART. Congestive headache, exploding from inside. Head heavy, pains into eyeballs. Sun headache. Blurry vision.

Ignatia—feels BAND AROUND HEAD, sighs, cries, lump in throat. Often from grief or stress breakdown. Nervous hysteria in women. Headache, as if a nail was driven into the side of the head. Right eye. From abuse of tobacco, alcohol, coffee, with nausea.

Iris versicolor—blindness, aura of colors (SPARKLY LIGHTS LIKE A RAINBOW) before the headache pain. Right side. Forehead right side. Throbbing, shooting. Headache from mental exhaustion. Alternates sides. Over one eye. With nausea, or low blood sugar symptoms.

Lachesis—headache upon waking. Left-sided. CAN'T STAND TIGHTNESS AROUND the neck. Talkative. Claustrophobic. Congestive rush of blood to the head. Throbbing or burning on the top of the head. Worse from sun, before menstruation, and in menopause. From abuse of alcohol. Mostly in women.

Lycopodium—right-sided headache. Liver involvement. Worse 4 to 8 P.M. With ravenous hunger. Better from eating, worse not eating. Pain in temples. Low self-esteem, worse after coughing, causes throbbing.

Nux-vomica—frontal right-sided headache. BRUISED BRAIN SENSATION. Nail in the top of the head. Mostly males, drinkers, use of stimulants. Liver and digestive problems—food sits in stomach like a rock. Toxic from alcohol, drugs. Hangover. Sunshine. Eyes sensitive to light.

Pulsatilla—WANDERING PAINS, in different areas of the head. Headache from overloaded stomach with pastry, fat, ice cream, or coffee. Worse walking in open air. Pulsating, bursting pains. Girls in puberty. Hormonal issues.

Sanguinaria—right-sided headache. From back of head over right eye. FLASH OF LIGHTNING PAINS. Veins in temples enlarged. Worse without food, and every seven days. Headaches from sunrise to the setting of the sun. Burning pains. Flushed face. Migraine headache remedy.

Silicea—Over one eye. Since a severe disease, top of head throbs. Pain, then visual disturbance. Worse with movement, noise, motion, light, cold air, and stools. Must keep head covered. Thin cold delicate shy people.

Spigelia—LEFT-SIDED headaches, pains and sinus, temple to eyes. THROBBING, violent, as if band around head. Worse stooping and opening the mouth. Migraine headache remedy.

HEARTBURN

Heartburn can happen with no symptoms at all, or there may be a sense of indigestion, or food can be coming up into the throat (reflux). The sensation is most often a warm or burning after eating, or at any time. A person may have to sit up in bed. Western medicine offers antacids to calm the acid reflux or burning sensation. They also frequently use proton pump inhibitors or PPIs, that stop stomach acid production—these are inherently dangerous as they can cause kidney damage, osteoporosis, anemia, etc., while never solving the underlying cause. However, the cause of heartburn is complex as the stomach, liver, gallbladder, pancreas, and small intestines are involved. It all starts typically with low stomach acid, then, when food is fermenting because it hasn't been broken down, an acid rebound happens causing heartburn (or reflux). Then the pancreatic enzymes will be ineffective, and the small intestines cannot absorb food efficiently. It disturbs our intestinal flora or microbiome where we produce 60 to 80 percent of our brain chemicals, affecting how we think and feel. Homeopathy offers great hope, when using the correct remedy.

Heartburn

Heartburn Story

Frequently, people come to see me in efforts to stop using their proton pump inhibitor drugs, with all their risks and side effects. Once, a man came to me complaining of heartburn, and food that seemed to sit in his stomach like a rock. He was a high-power businessman who used alcohol, stimulants, energy drinks, and PPI drugs to cope with stress. I suggested Nux Vomica 200C once a week. A few weeks later he reported that he was coping with stress much better, had no more heartburn, and felt less desire for alcohol and stimulants.

Heartburn Essential Remedies

Arsenicum album—with BURNING SENSATION in the throat. Heartburn worse from vinegar, ice cream, and ice water (which can cause immediate vomiting). Worse from 10 P.M. to 2 A.M. The perfectionist. This remedy also works for food poisoning.

Calc carb—heartburn with frequent SOUR BELCHING or vomiting after eating. Water causes nausea. With obesity and weak ankles. Useful in children and during pregnancy.

Carbo veg—heartburn with gas and BELCHING THAT RELIEVES. Stomach feels empty, can't even think about food. Stomach cramping from excess gas. Gas is sour or putrid.

Conium—heartburn that is WORSE AFTER MILK. Bloating, sick feeling, acidity, belching. The sternum (chest) is painful. Feels worse going to bed.

Lycopodium—bloating with pressure on the lungs, worse 4 to 8 P.M. Heartburn rises to the throat. Worse after eating, mornings, sweets, cabbage, BEANS, onions, pastries. Feels full after a little food.

Nux vomica—food sits like a rock in the stomach. Ravenous appetite. HEARTBURN FROM OVEREATING, must loosen belt. More in males who abuse alcohol and stimulants.

Phosphorus—heartburn with EMPTY FEELING IN STOMACH. Cold stomach, hangs down. Sour taste and belching after meals. Cold food or drink causes vomiting. Social, sensitive.

HEMORRHOIDS

Symptoms of hemorrhoids include pain mostly in the anal region with redness and possible bulging hemorrhoid. Hemorrhoids can be single or like a bunch of grapes—they can protrude out of the anus or be internal. Pain usually starts from a bowel movement. Pain can also come from merely walking. Causes from a poor diet or nutrition, or from the liver that can no longer remove bodily toxins effectively—the portal vein from the liver, which goes to the anus, may become weakened and create hemorrhoids. Western medicine may use topical pain relievers or surgically remove the hemorrhoids. Natural methods such as homeopathy, specifically, can help the liver to function better and to help eliminate the hemorrhoids.

Hemorrhoid Story
Hemorrhoids are not a favorite subject of mine, but a frequent concern of my clients. A grumpy woman came to see me complaining of hemorrhoids that felt like slivers were stuck in the anus, as well as having fissures (deep skin cracks). She tried Nitric Acid 30C, two pellets three times a day, as suggested. She came back in a month, much more pleasant—sticking pains were gone, and the anal fissures were clearing up.

Hemorrhoid Essential Remedies
Aesculus Hipp—BURNING ANUS, chills go up and down the back. Pains from stools. Hemorrhoids with sharp shooting pains, internal hemorrhoids that cause bleeding, purple and painful. External. Worse walking and standing, and during menopause. Itching, chronic, burning, from wiping.

Hemorrhoids

Arsenicum album—HEMORRHOIDS BURN LIKE FIRE. Better by heat. Burning pains and pressure, caused from alcohol. Itching, red, sore, external. Large hemorrhoids. Worse walking. The perfectionist. Worse 10 P.M. to 2 A.M.

Carbo veg—bluish burning painful hemorrhoids, worse after stools, worse alcohol. ITCHING. Chronic. External hemorrhoids are large. Poor digestion, gas and bloating.

Causticum—hemorrhoids chronic, external, very itchy and large, worse walking. Wants justice.

Hamamelis—hemorrhoids BLEED PROFUSELY and are sore. Painful hard stools. Large external hemorrhoids that burn, often chronic. Blue, painful, itching, external, sore, bruised sensation.

Lachesis—hemorrhoids purple and protruding. Sharp pains on coughing or sneezing. Chronic, external, painful. Hemorrhoids worse menstruation, or menopause. Worse alcohol. Mostly females. Jealous, strong emotions.

Nitric Acid—anal fissures (deep cracks in skin). Violent cutting pains. Hemorrhages if hemorrhoids are surgically removed. HEMORRHOIDS BLEED EASILY, sharp stitching pains. Large, painful, internal hemorrhoids, worse on walking. Grumpy person.

Nux vomica—hemorrhoids INTERNAL, burning, chronic. Large with constipation and digestive problems (liver). Burning and painful. Mostly males who crave alcohol or stimulants. High-powered businessmen. Worse or caused by alcohol.

Sulphur—anal redness, stool smells like rotten eggs. HEMORRHOIDS OOZING, external and internal, large, sore, tender, raw, burning, bleeding, blue, chronic. Worse walking and wiping. The intellectual disorganized person.

HOT FLASHES

Hot flash symptoms usually come in the menopausal years of women ages 49 plus, although some come much earlier for those with medical menopause (hysterectomy). These may come earlier or later. Hot flashes consist of an uncontrollable, uncomfortable, warm sensation lasting minutes to hours, with or without profuse sweating causing a need to change clothes. They can come on randomly, or at night only. Causation is the natural changes of menopause or hormonal imbalances if younger. The body is changing and hormonal production shifts from the ovaries to the adrenal glands and liver. This change may trigger the hypothalamus to dysregulate metabolism and temperature control. Western medicine uses hormone replacement or "bioidentical" hormone drugs, so called, to contain symptoms, but they are not natural at all. While there are risks or toxicity, this may create a lifetime dependency. Homeopathy can help the body to transition to normal post-menopausal function.

Hot Flash Story
Hot flashes are a very frequent complaint in peri-menopausal and menopausal women, from younger women even to women in their nineties. A woman came to see me in her early fifties complaining of weight gain, low sex drive, persistent hot flashes, and feeling disconnected from her children and husband. Using Sepia 30C, two pellets three times a day—and a month later—most of her complaints were resolved.

Hot Flash Essential Remedies

Cimicifuga—uterine prolapse. PAINS IN NECK, SHOULDER, across hips. Feels as if a black cloud is hanging over. Dejected. Lots of fears. Hypochondriac.

Lachesis—can be bipolar, can't stand anything tight on around the neck. Claustrophobic. Sweaty HOT FLASHES AT NIGHT. High sex drive. Heart palpitations. Prolapsed uterus. Headaches. Heat in the head.

Sepia—hormonal changes in menopause with weight gain. Wants to be alone. Low sex drive. #1 remedy for uterine prolapse. Painful sex. DRY VAGINA. Sudden hot flashes.

Calc Carb—tendency to obesity. Family person. Weak ankles. Cold damp feet. HOT FLASHES WITH SWEAT.

Graphites—tendency to OBESITY AND ECZEMA. Keloid scars. Low sex drive.

Pulsatilla—PEOPLE-PLEASERS. High sex drive. Emotional, sweating from hot flashes. Whiny, cries easily.

HYPOGLYCEMIA (LOW BLOOD SUGAR)

Blood sugar (glucose) drops at times, which can cause anxiety, anxiousness, irritability, nervous instability or severe fatigue. There may also be cold sweats, shaking, and heart palpitations. Often the cause is a poor diet, rich in sugars, or frequent fast food with sugar-rich sodas. If guilty, change your diet! Western medicine contributes; in their treatment of common diseases or ailments, they interfere with digestion using antacids and PPIs (proton pump inhibitors) that create digestive dysregulation, toxicity, and side effects. Basic digestion requires sufficient stomach acid, helping the pancreas to release sodium bicarb to maintain the correct acid alkaline balance or pH, so the small intestine can utilize the pancreatic enzymes to break the food down properly. The liver is also involved as it stores sugar, or glycogen, to be released at the proper time to maintain proper insulin and sugar levels in the blood. Homeopathy offers help—as a person's symptoms match the homeopathic remedies to help correct underlying weaknesses.

Hypoglycemia Story
Hypoglycemia is usually secondary to other health issues and the right homeopathic can help an underlying cause. A thin, hyperactive, teenage man came to me complaining that he couldn't gain any weight. He

was nervous and had a huge appetite. I suggested Iodum 30C, once a day. A month later he came back, more calm and focused, had gained a couple of pounds and was happier about his weight.

Hypoglycemia Essential Remedies

Graphites—NEEDS TO EAT FREQUENTLY. Obesity. Skin issues. Scars easily. Sweats easily.

Iodium*—thyroid overactive. Emaciation. BIG APPETITE, LOSES WEIGHT. Hyperactive.

Kali Carb obesity. Worse during the night 2 to 4 A.M. Duty-bound people.

Lycopodium—low self-esteem. All symptoms worse 4 to 8 P.M. Liver weakness. Pancreas weakness.

Phosphorus—Distracted from eating regularly. Others energy affects them. Sensitive.

Silicea—EMACIATION. General weakness. COLD, TIMID, weak.

Sulphur—OVERHEATED. Intellectual and skin problems.

*Not in Materia Medica. Not common.

INCONTINENCE

Those with symptoms of incontinence have leaky urine at random times—when they laugh, walk, jump, or cough—requiring them to wear absorptive pads. Found mostly in women, the cause comes from having babies, also happening in menopause with low estrogen causing pelvic tissue weakness, and urinary valve weakness. Homeopathy can help the body correct hormonal and tissue weakness. Western medicine drugs dry up urinary leakage. One of the side effects is cognitive decline (brain fog), dependency on the drug, and toxicity.

Incontinence

Incontinence Story

I have consulted with many women regarding their incontinence, especially after childbirth. They leak from physical activity, coughing, or laughing. Most of the time Causticum 30C, at two pellets twice a day, will produce less significant leakage in a week or less, and permanent results in two to three months.

Incontinence Essential Remedies

Apis Mel—"Queen bee." INCONTINENCE FROM UTIs with stinging and burning. Involuntary passing of urine, feels hot. Worse coughing. Often in elderly.

Argentum Nit—URINE PASSES UNKNOWN, night or day. Worse from fears, being in groups of people. Often in the elderly. "Fear of performance" and heights. Panic attacks. Claustrophobia. Craves sugar or chocolates.

Arsenicum album—incontinence from childbirth. INVOLUNTARY BURNING, may have a bad smell. Often in ELDERLY. Worse 10 P.M. to 2 A.M. "Perfectionist."

Belladonna—profuse urination. Acute inflammation. Sudden, violent. Red face, throbbing pains. INCONTINENCE FROM CHILDBIRTH. Worse night, lying or standing, coughing, or when sleeping during the day. "Expressing anger."

Causticum—#1 remedy for incontinence. Urine dribbles, passes better when sitting. From childbirth. COUGHING, LAUGHING, walking, sneezing, excitement. From childbirth. "Advocate for justice" personality.

Lycopodium—profuse URINATION AT NIGHT. Involuntary urination from fevers or bad dreams. Aching in right kidney. Coughing. Everything worse 4 to 8 P.M. "Low self-esteem," is often bullied.

Nat Mur—SUDDEN NEED TO URINATE. Urinate while coughing, laughing, sneezing, or walking. Can't urinate when others are around. Dryness of skin, and lips. "Introvert" from emotional hurts. Craves salt.

Pulsatilla—dribbling when angry. UNCONSCIOUS URINATION AT NIGHT, during sleep, and when coughing, sneezing, laughing, passing gas, sudden noises, surprises, shocks. "Shy, clingy, people pleaser."

Sepia—everything worse from HORMONAL CHANGES. Childbirth, menstruation, menopause, coughing, or laughing. "Introverted and sensitive."

INJURIES, *see also*: HEAD INJURIES

Injuries happen—all types, including falls, blows, tears, cuts and more. Several types of pain are associated with injuries, along with bruising, tissue damage, swelling, redness, and bleeding. Homeopathic medicine can be spectacular for injuries—used best when the injury just happened. The results can be fast, at time of injury, and improvements can continue in days, weeks and months or years later. "Emergency" or "Injury" remedies work remarkably fast when used right at the time or after the injury has happened. They can be more effective than over-the-counter or prescription pain medications. Emergency injuries usually require 200C potency, frequently used to contain pain and damage. Use of a 30C potency can be used, but pain-relieving effects wear off faster. First-aid homeopathics are remarkable for their ability to facilitate reduction in pain, bleeding and also in promoting faster healing.

Injuries Story
A young woman smashed her fingers in a car door. Her mom was quick to use Hypericum 200C, for nerve damage and nerve pain, and the pain subsided within minutes. This is typical of results with First-Aid homeopathics.

Injuries Essential Remedies

Arnica—#1 remedy for ALL INJURIES. Use Arnica first for all injuries in a 30 C or 200C, several times as needed. SOFT TISSUE INJURIES from blows, contusions. Injury from overexertion. Limping. Use before and after playing sports or exercise. Bed feels too hard. Better stretching, worse touch.

Bellis perennis—SWELLING. Injuries from blows with swelling, bruising. Nerve pains. Soreness. Bruised aching. Hip pain. Better continued motion (Rhus Tox), cold compresses and pressure. Worse lifting, before storms. Use when Arnica no longer works.

Bryonia—SHARP PAINS UPON MOVEMENT. Joints are red, hot and swollen. Weak knees. Pains better from warmth. For blows, soreness, and limping.

Cantharis—#1 remedy for BURNS (first- and second-degree). Burning pains with blisters and redness. Also burning in UTIs.

Staphysagria—#1 remedy for SURGICAL CUTS. Sharp cuts.

Hypericum—#1 remedy for NERVE PAINS (RADIATING). Spinal or coccyx(tailbone) injuries. Worse bites, stings, cuts-surgery, cold damp, touch, pressure, storms, night. Better rubbing, lying down quietly. From blows, nerve injuries, or neuralgia.

Nat Sulph—#1 remedy for HEAD INJURIES. Mental and physical problems. Depression, headaches. From blows to the head. Head injury after-effects. Worse cold damp places or weather, and night. Better dry warm air, movement, pressure.

Rhus Tox—#1 remedy for JOINT INJURIES worse from first movement, better from continued motion. Stiffness. Cracking joints. Tearing pains in tendons, ligaments, tissues, sciatica, numbness, and prickling. Ankles or knees swollen. Worse cold damp and stormy weather.

Ruta Grav—#1 remedy for TENDON INJURIES—worse from overactivity, lifting, sprains, injuries. Ganglion cyst. Hamstring injury. Thighs feel broken. Tendonitis, sciatica, and limping from blows. Soreness. Better from warmth.

Symphytum—#1 remedy for BONE INJURIES. Bone fractures, prickling pain. PERIOSTEUM injury. Non-union fracture, osteoporosis. Better warmth, worse touch, motion, pressure. From blunt trauma injury.

ITCHING

When the skin is either too dry, becomes red, or is burning, we itch. There may be itching with or without pain, or biting sensation (sharp pain). Itches may, or may not, come with rashes, bleeding or fissures (deep cracks in skin). The itching can feel better from heat or cold. It may cause sleeplessness. In my experience, 90 percent of the time the itching or other skin conditions are a result of liver imbalance, and sometimes kidney imbalance. Liver symptoms include irritability, anger, waking from 2 to 4 A.M., waking up tired, and of course having skin problems. Liver imbalance usually comes from alcohol damage, sometimes more than one drink a day, or the person cannot tolerate alcohol or caffeine. Other major liver challenges come from over-the-counter and prescription medications, some cause more liver damage than others. The homeopathic remedies often help the body improve the liver, and then skin function. Western medicine recommends steroid cream use that sometimes helps symptoms, but may cause lung damage and are ultimately toxic.

Itching Story
A mother brought in her "incorrigible child" to see me. The child fit the Sulphur remedy in personality, and a history of skin issues suppressed by steroid creams. One dose of Sulphur found her "darling happy child" returned. But, in a few days, the wet itching eczema returned to his

face. She put on the steroid creams again, and the "incorrigible child" returned as soon as the skin condition was suppressed by the cream. Her response was that the eczema looked worse than the child's terrible behavior!

Itching Essential Remedies

Causticum—itching with rash, burning, must scratch. ITCHING AND ECZEMA IN FOLDS OF SKIN, back of ears, between thighs. Worse in good weather, dry cold air, wind or draft, 3 A.M., and from 6 to 8 P.M. Better in damp wet weather, washing, and warmth.

Mezereum—Rash, biting (sharp pain), burning, intolerable itching. ERUPTIONS HAVE YELLOW DISCHARGE, crust over, pus underneath. Itching in the elderly. All symptoms worse at night, warmth of bed, cold air, draft. Better in open air and wrapping up.

Petroleum—ITCHING ECZEMA WITH CRACKS in skin. Must scratch. Psoriasis on hands. Deep cracks in skin folds. Cracks bleed easily. Skin hard, rough, thickened, pus under greenish crusts, burning, itching. Worse dampness, cold, WINTER, changing weather. Better warm, dry.

Rhus Tox—itching associated with arthritis. INTENSE ITCHING. Poison ivy. Herpes. Rashes. Burning after scratching worse with rubbing. Boils, abscesses. Feels better in hot water. Worse storms, cold damp weather. Better heat.

Sulphur—#1 remedy for skin issues. Burning, especially symptoms when scratching. CRACKS, ECZEMA, ULCERS. Unhealthy skin. Injuries cause pus. Worse in folds of skin. Worse bathing, warmth, morning around 11 A.M., at night, storms, alcohol, and the full moon. Better dry warm weather.

LEG ULCERS

Leg ulcers include symptoms of discoloration of the lower legs, weakness of the lower legs. These may proceed to open sores that may not heal easily, then to weeping fluids. In the worst cases, let ulcers may result in gangrene and loss of legs. Leg ulcers happen more often in the elderly, and diabetic patients. Causations include: weakness of the veins and arteries that may leak or bleed, or loss of circulation; injury; circulatory problem with either or both legs; smoking. Homeopathy can be great help, along with medications.

Leg Ulcer Story

Leg ulcers come on gradually and are usually found in the elderly. To reach a satisfactory result will require a close homeopathic symptom match. Homeopathic treatment works at a 30C potency, two pellets three times a day for several months with measurable and gradual results.

Leg Ulcer Remedies

Arsenicum album—leg ulcers that have a black base with SURROUNDING BLUISH TISSUE. There can be burning discharges with nerve pains and may progress to diabetic gangrene. The perfectionist. Worse 10 P.M. to 2 A.M.

Carbo Veg—the ULCERS HAVE A BLACK BASE, are painful, mottled, with skin around or surrounding tissue that can bleed. Bad-smelling discharges. There is swelling, burning, cold legs. Legs seem to go to sleep. People with heart problems. Digestive issues, gas.

Lachesis—the SURROUNDING TISSUE MOTTLED BLUE, sensitive to touch, bloody smelly discharges. It is a black base, purple tissue, better from bleeding. Can progress to gangrene. Worse during menstruation or during menopause. Mostly in intense women, mostly left-sided.

Lycopodium—leg ulcers have a black base, burning and ITCHING, VERY PAINFUL. Limbs go to sleep. It may progress to gangrene. Symptoms are worse 4 to 8 P.M. Mostly right-sided.

MACULAR DEGENERATION

Affecting eyesight, deterioration or degeneration of the macula takes away center vision, leaving only peripheral (outer) vision. Reading or other activities may be difficult. Causation of macular degeneration is a bit of a theory—that blood supply and circulation are most important and may be compromised—from a poor diet, drugs, or especially from smoking. It may be a result of lack of antioxidants. Western medicine likely recommends antioxidants, which mostly work to stop the progression. Homeopathy offers some help to stabilize or improve vision.

Macular Degeneration Story
Carboneum Sulph is a little-used homeopathic remedy, but I have seen it work to RESTORE CENTRAL VISION in several people. I don't use this remedy for much else, although it works on other eye symptoms. Vision is precious. Use the 30C, two pellets three times a day. The changes are gradual over several months.

Macular Degeneration Essential Remedies

Apis Mel—obscured (VEIL OVER EYES SENSATION) or weak vision, gray mist. Near-sighted. Objects look too large. Allergic puffy eyelids. Hot tears, sudden sharp pains. Indistinct vision. Squinting. Vision is better with stool. Causation allergic reactions.

Bovista—TENDENCY TO BLEEDING in the eyes. Causation from carbon monoxide poisoning. Vision week and dim. Mucus in eyes at night. Pressure in eye sensation. Objects look nearer than they are. Retinal paralysis. Vision only on one side vertically.

Carboneum sulph—nearsighted. CENTRAL VISION LOSS. Dim vision. Vision that objects fade away in a fog. Color blindness. Nervous system weakness. Causation—carbon monoxide poisoning. Vision better evenings after eating.

Calc Ars—Pain in right eye. LETTERS LOOK TO RUN TOGETHER. Obesity. Anxiety, restlessness.

Gelsemium—Pain above eyes even after correct glasses. Vision slow to accommodate. WORDS DIM, RUN TOGETHER. Worse stooping. Blindness with dilated pupils. Double vision looking sideways. M.S., headache. Vision affected by masturbation. Worse distant vision. Affects the nervous system, panic attacks. Causation—shock, alcohol, drugs.

Lachesis—Can't focus, flickering vision. GLITTERING VISION (sparkly lights like a rainbow). Blindness with lung or heart problems. Causation—injuries, stress of being caretakers, disappointed love, alcoholism. Rapid rambling speech. Often seen in people with BIPOLAR disorder.

Phosphorus—Retina problems, narrow vision. Double vision. SEES A GREEN HALO. Misty vision. Letters look red. Vision loss from tobacco, too much sex, or lightning. Causation—emotions, electricity. Oversensitivity, can't focus.

Sepia—Black spots or points. Contracted pupils. SEES SPARKS OR FLASHES. Vision changes with menstruation. Vision affected by masturbation, hormonal or sexual excesses. Cause—hormonal changes. Mostly seen in women.

MENOPAUSE

When a woman's reproductive hormones start to wane, she goes into perimenopause. Menopause, defined, is when a woman has not menstruated for 12 months. Hormonal production during perimenopause shifts from the ovaries to the adrenal glands and liver. When the adrenal glands are functioning in a healthy way, the body produces all the hormones needed so that the aging signs of low estrogen are minimized (skin wrinkles, breasts sagging, vaginal dryness, hot flashes). Symptoms of hormonal health include staying happy (emotionally), keeping a good memory, and sleeping well. Other factors of hormonal imbalances include thyroid health, losing hair on the head and growing excess hair on the face (hirsutism). Several homeopathic remedies can be helpful to prevent challenges or enhance overall help for a gentle transition and vibrant life as we age. Vaginal dryness can be soothed by calendula cream used vaginally, and evening primrose oil consumed internally.

Menopause Story
I consulted with a menopausal woman who complained of a low sex drive, and an inability to connect with her family emotionally. She often yelled at them and retreated into her room. This happened at age 50 when she entered menopause. The remedy Sepia, taken for two weeks, helped her find connection with her children, and raised her sex drive with her husband.

Menopause Essential Remedies

Cimicifuga—fear of insanity, BLACK CLOUD OF DEPRESSION OVERHEAD. Pain of neck and shoulders hormonal. Tendency to obesity. Pale, anxious, restless. Vision problems, dizziness in menopause with nerve pains or arthritis.

Lachesis—nervous, talkative, jumps from one subject to another. Can't stand any clothing tight, especially around the neck. High sex drive. Hot flashes, SWEATY AT NIGHT, heat in head, hair loss, headaches. Depressed at night. Feels worse upon waking. Intense person. Can be bipolar or alcoholic.

Sepia—sweaty, hot flashes. Headaches. #1 remedy for HAIR LOSS. Dark circles under the eyes. Yellow skin. #1 remedy for hirsutism (DARK, THICK, COARSE HAIR ON FACE). Weak thyroid. Obesity. Osteoporosis. Breast and uterine fibroids. Incontinence. LOW SEX DRIVE. Vaginal dryness, discharges, feels like uterus will fall out. Must exercise to feel good. Often intuitive. INTROVERTED. Feels worse when consoled.

Calc carb—OBESITY. Breast fibroids, fatigue, hair loss, thyroid issues, osteoporosis, CONSTIPATION. Vaginal dryness, discharges. Weak ankles. Home body. Lots of fears. Wants CONSOLATION.

Graphites—DOUBTS SELF, weeping. Hair loss, hot flashes, vaginal dryness and discharges, uterine fibroids. OBESITY. LOW SEX DRIVE. SKIN problems. Scars easily, eczema with yellow honey-like discharges.

Nat Mur—INTROVERT, depression, grief, cries only in private. Worse from consolation. DRYNESS in tissues or thin clear abundant mucus. Extreme vaginal dryness. Incontinence. Hair falls out when touched, excess facial hair (hirsutism). Thyroid weakness. Uterine fibroids. Low sex drive due to vaginal dryness and emotional issues. Craves salt.

Pulsatilla—PEOPLE PLEASER, hard to make decisions. Cries easily, weepy and whiny. Fears of abandonment. Hot flashes sweaty. Higher sex drive when not painful. Bland changeable discharges, vaginal dryness. Breast fibroids, uterine polyps. Hair falls out. Incontinence. Can't tolerate fats (gallbladder issues).

MENSTRUAL ISSUES

Hormones, for women, are constantly changing throughout the month. This can bring on anything from irritability, tension, anxiety, mood swings, or depression, to sex-drive changes, and crying. Physically, there may be pain, cramping, bleeding, acne, and bloating during times of the month. Causes of hormonal imbalances may be inherited weaknesses, chemical toxicity, dietary indiscretions, smoking, excess alcohol, or other stimulants or drugs. Xeno-estrogens (foreign) disrupt hormone functioning. Stress and injuries also contribute. The worst culprit to hormone imbalances is chemical birth control—many women are never well since using it. Homeopathic remedies can help the body to correct these hormonal imbalance symptom patterns—mental as well as physical. *See also* PMS.

Menstrual Issues Story
A woman in her mid-30s came to me complaining of being overly emotional, with symptoms changing all the time. She had a fear of abandonment. A week after taking Pulsatilla, she felt more emotionally in control with less weeping. Physically, she was more stable with less pain or cramping.

Menstrual Issues Essential Remedies

Cimicifuga—menstruation with depression as if a dark cloud hanging over, with neck and shoulder pain. Nerve pains with menstruation. BACKACHE, THE MORE FLOW THE MORE PAIN, with hip to hip pain as well, and cramping ovarian nerve pain.

Colocynthis—menstruation with SCREAMING PAINS, must double over. Flow is copious and too frequent. Ovarian cysts. Worse anger with indignation (taking offense).

Mag Phos—menstruation with CRAMPING PAINS. Nerve pains. The flow is too early. Flows at night. Worse from noise, excitement. Better from walking, heat, and bending over.

Sepia–irregular, early, profuse menstruation, or late and scanty menstruation. Uterine congestion. Nerve pains, PAIN IN THIGHS. Tall and thin person, or obese. Left-sided ovarian pain. Low sex drive, wants to be alone.

Belladonna—menstruation with inflammation, right sided, THROBBING PAINS. Cramping pains that are bearing down with right-sided ovarian pains. Menses too early, bright red blood.

Ignatia—menstruation suppressed from grief. Stopped menstruation, or too early or profuse with black bloody clots. Pain with pressure. EMOTIONAL, LUMP IN THROAT.

Kali Carb—PMS with SWOLLEN BREASTS, and water retention. Menstruation is smelly, with violent colic. Obesity with black and white thinking. Worse after childbirth. Pain goes down the thighs.

Pulsatilla—menstruation has CHANGEABLE SYMPTOMS, pains are crampy with nerve pain. Menstruation too late, scanty, or irregular. Emotional, abandonment issues. Worse at puberty. Weepy, wants to be consoled.

MONONUCLEOSIS

Symptoms of mononucleosis include extreme fatigue and sometimes swollen lymph glands, or a swollen spleen, which can last a few weeks to the rest of your life. Western medicine has no answers. The chronic form of mononucleosis can be the Epstein-Barr virus, or turn into Chronic Fatigue Syndrome. Causation is often called the "kissing disease," resembles cytomegalovirus, is saliva- and air-borne. Your immune system determines how you are affected. Homeopathic therapies, in my experience, can shorten the effects of the virus. I have seen results in just a few days.

Mononucleosis Story
A sixteen-year-old had mononucleosis for eight months and lost a year of attending school. I suggested twenty-five drops of Ceanothus* tincture, three times a day in a little water, and Mercury Sol 30C, two pellets three times a day. She returned to school in five days.

Mononucleosis Essential Remedies

Calc carb—longstanding health issues, chronic fatigue and weakness. OBESITY. WEAK ANKLES, loose joints. Overwork.

Carcinosin—acute symptoms, CHRONIC FATIGUE AND CHRONIC WEAKNESS. Tired and weak, over organized person. Longstanding health issues.

Gelsemium—used to prevent mono. Ailments from mononucleosis, chronic fatigue and weakness. INTERNAL SHAKING, apathy, feeling wiped out, dull, heavy limbs. No thirst.

Mercury Sol or Vivus—#1 remedy for mononucleosis, in my experience. Acute or chronic mononucleosis. Recent or longstanding illnesses. Chronic fatigue and weakness. TIRED AND WEAK, sweaty, sore throat, chills, mouth ulcers, tonsil abscess.

Ceanothus*—25 drops of mother-tincture dose in a little water three times a day. Also works in chronic, post mononucleosis symptoms. (Between Mercury Sol and Ceanothus*, the body responds in less than a week.) Also called Red Root.

*Not in Materia Medica. Not common.

MORNING SICKNESS

Women can experience nausea and/or vomiting during pregnancy from food (with or without eating) or smells, and anytime of the day or night. Morning sickness can be severe and debilitating. Causes are usually hormonal changes in the beginning, and the stomach getting squeezed in later pregnancy. Western pharmaceutical drugs always have some risks, but may be necessary in rare cases. Homeopathy can help the body overcome nausea and vomiting and is absolutely safe during pregnancy. See also Nausea and Vomiting.

Morning Sickness Story
A woman who worked for me was in her first trimester of pregnancy. She became deathly nauseated and vomited frequently. No Western drugs seem to help. Each day, for five days, we tried a different homeopathic remedy to no avail. And although I don't remember the exact one, on the sixth day we tried another remedy and it worked—she felt normal within a couple of hours of taking the remedy and stayed that way!

Morning Sickness Essential Remedies

Ipecac—#1 remedy for morning sickness. HAS A CLEAN TONGUE. Persistent nausea with a hanging down stomach sensation and cramping, rumbling, salivation, dry heaves. Throws up blood or food or watery liquids.

Lactic Acid —painful muscles, burning weight in stomach with hot acrid belching. PALE ANEMIC women. Constant nausea, better from eating, worse from smelling smoke.

Mercury Sol—with EXCESS DROOLING, nausea and vomiting while coughing, at stool. Vomiting bile and food. Has changeable emotions.

Nux Vomica—FOOD SITS LIKE A ROCK IN THE STOMACH. Sour taste with nausea in the morning, hiccups from overeating. Stomach feels heavy, painful, sensitive to pressure, must loosen clothes. Irritability.

Pulsatilla—bitter taste or diminished taste. Stomach feels heavy, gassy, FROM FATTY FOODS. Vomits after eating fruits. Pale face, feels chilly, better in fresh air. Weeping, whiny people-pleasers.

Sepia—stomach has sinking feeling or burning in pit of stomach. Stomach feels empty. Feels worse from bread, milk, and fats. NAUSEA AT THE THOUGHT OR SMELL OF FOOD. Vomiting of milk fluid, bile, and food. Introverts, want to be alone, no sex drive.

MUCUS

Secretions from the mucus membranes can be thin or thick, watery. They may have a taste, or not. We usually think of mucus when it is over-produced and becomes an inconvenience or a problem. The body over-produces mucus for a good reason. It is a sign of what is going on inside the body. The least problematic mucus is clear, then goes to

Mucus

thicker, white, yellow, then green, then brown, or even black (dried blood—more serious, or deeper issue). Causes of mucus are many: the body uses mucus to envelop toxicity, dust, and more, and push it out. It is a natural process. Excess mucus is often caused by poor digestion, which can then move from the digestive tract into the sinuses, lungs, and can appear in the stools. When a condition or disease is getting better the mucus production and colors become lighter and thinner. Western drugs, antibiotics, can kill invading bacteria but may only make the problem worse by not dealing with the underlying cause. Homeopathy can help the underlying cause to minimize excess mucus. Each homeopathic remedy may encourage mucus to progress to different colors, or you may have to respond with a different remedy at a stage of mucus color change. Pay attention to symptoms from the Keynotes in the Remedy chapter (Materia Medica). The better the match, the better the results.

Mucus Story

A woman came to consult with me for excess mucus in her stools, which she had observed for several months. She didn't feel "quite right." The mucus changed frequently in color and consistency. I suggested the remedy Pulsatilla. She took it daily and it cleared up in less than a month.

Mucus Essential Remedies

Arsenicum album—mucus is yellow, green, brown, thin. Burning discharges, better from heat. Perfectionist. Worse 10 P.M. to 2 A.M.

Belladonna—mucus is thin, bloody, white or yellow. Fever, or throbbing pain. Irritable.

Carbo veg—mucus is thin, bloody, yellow, green, or brown. GASSY person.

Hydrastis*—mucus is YELLOW, THICK, ROPY, raw, irritating, and burning. Apathetic from debilitating disease.

Kali Bich—mucus is yellow or green, THICK AND STRINGY. Impatient person. Frequently in children.

Kreosotum—mucus is BLOODY, all colors, mostly yellow, green. Irritating, hot, BAD-SMELLING discharges, to gangrene. Tissue breakdown. Person irritable, denies they have a problem.

Mercury Sol—mucus is watery and thin, bloody, white, yellow, green. Pus formation, SMELLS BAD. Can't make up their mind.

Nat Mur—mucus copious clear watery, and SALTY. Dry person, craves salt. Introvert.

Nitric Acid—mucus is thin, bloody, YELLOW OR GREEN, IRRITATING and thin, Decay products, causing redness. Splinter pains. Pessimistic.

Phosphorus—mucus is bloody, white, yellow, or green. SENSITIVE person, extrovert.

Pulsatilla—mucus is CHANGEABLE, smooth, white to yellow. Weepy, whiny people-pleasers. Mostly in women.

Sepia—mucus is bloody, white, yellow, green, thick. SENSITIVE TO ODORS. Introvert, sensitive person. Hormonal problems. Mostly in women.

Silicea—mucus is bloody, thin, white, yellow, green, with pus production. Thin, shy and delicate cold person. Sears easily.

*Not in Materia Medica. Not common.

MUSCLE CRAMPS

Cramping pain can come on suddenly or gradually, during the day or only at night. It can last for several seconds, or minutes. Pain can be short-lived, or last long after the actual cramps subside. Causes of muscle cramps are usually physical exertion, sweating out minerals such as magnesium, calcium, or potassium. If you don't consume enough minerals or are taking PPIs (proton pump inhibitor) drugs, which lower stomach acid and limit absorption of vitamins and especially minerals, you may get muscle cramps. Homeopathy can help with muscle cramps, relief comes sometimes in seconds. For those who get cramps at night, take your homeopathic remedy before bed.

Muscle Cramps Story
I have innumerable elderly people who complain of nightly leg cramps that disturb their sleep, with pain. Nightly left-leg cramps are almost always prevented by using Cuprum Met. There are a lot of grateful people!

Muscle Cramps Essential Remedies

Top three remedies:

Calc carb—weak ankles, trembling, weakness, CLUMSY person, sweaty hands, tendency to obesity. Calf cramps, cold damp feet. Mostly right sided.

Cuprum met—calf cramps, soles, palms, fingers, and toes. Worse especially at night, from pressure, cold, hot weather. More left sided.

Mag phos—spasms and stiffness of limbs, clenched. Fingers and thumbs, worse at night and in bed. CRAMPS IN CALVES AND IN FEET. Writer's and runner's cramps. Pregnancy cramps. Phantom limb pain. Better from heat, doubling over, exhaustion, touch. More right-sided.

Other muscle cramp remedies:

Arnica—cramping from an INJURY, sore bruise sensation. Over exercise. No particular side. Finger cramps, writer's cramp, loss of muscle strength.

Belladonna—THROBBING AND CRAMPING pain. Muscle spasms, cramps of limbs, limbs feel cold. Right sided.

Kali brom—caused by emotional stress. WRIST, HANDS, FINGERS IN CONSTANT MOTION. Worse at night, 2 A.M, hot weather. Trembling hands. No particular side.

Nux vomica—more males from overworked and using stimulants with digestive problems. Alcoholism. Cramps of limbs, calves, soles of the feet. LIMBS FEEL HEAVY. More right sided.

Veratrum album—caused by injury or stimulant abuse. CRAMPS IN CALVES DURING STOOL. Sciatica with electrical pains. Abdominal problems. More right sided.

Zinc met—slightly more left sided. Causation is concussion or emotional challenges. RESTLESS LEG syndrome. Worse from 5 to 7 P.M. Restless feet, trembling, twitching. Cramps, twitching of hands and feet.

NAUSEA AND VOMITING

Nausea and/or vomiting is the body's response to a perceived toxin that needs to be thrown up and out of the body. Sometimes it can be merely a smell that starts it. It can trigger the stomach muscles to cramp. Several organs including the stomach, liver, gallbladder, pancreas, and small intestine can be involved. Nausea can come from a myriad of problems, mostly from digestive issues. It is one of the body's defense mechanisms for protection against food poisoning. It can also come from emotional responses to perceived danger, or reminders of past traumas. There are food triggers, and also smell triggers, consciously or subconsciously. Pregnancy often causes this mechanism for unknown reasons (*see also* Morning Sickness). Western medications have anti-emetics, but those have side effects and may not address the underlying problem. Homeopathy can provide some real answers and usually will work very quickly. Homeopathics need only be chosen to match the symptoms and may give immediate results or, if symptoms are longstanding, attain gradual results.

Nausea and Vomiting Story

Many mothers come to me to help their children with nausea and vomiting, due to poorly diagnosed stomach issues, and Western drugs haven't helped or given bad side effects, worse than the nausea and vomiting. Homeopathic Ipecac works with quick and gratifying results—it tends to work most of the time. If it fails in a week's time, try other remedies.

Nausea and Vomiting Essential Remedies

Lobelia—SALIVATION WITH ASTHMA. PREGNANCY. With anxiety, headaches, after eating, in the sleep, with salivation.

Nux vomica—food sits in the stomach like a rock. PREGNANCY—1st or 2nd remedy to use. Nausea and vomiting that is painful. Anxiety and irritability with salivation. Worse after eating. Constant nausea from fever. Seasickness. Angry and irritable person. Stimulant or alcohol cravings.

Tabaccum—DEATHLY SICK at the pit of the stomach. #1 remedy for nausea and vomiting. SEASICKNESS. PREGNANCY, severe nausea and vomiting. Nausea worse from smoking. Worse with noise with an anxiety. Nausea with headaches.

Cocculus indicus—with VERTIGO from motion, light, noise, cold, constipation, drinking, after eating, SMELLS, afternoons, with headaches. SALIVA and sour, bitter taste when vomiting. PREGNANCY. TRAVEL SICKNESS (motion).

Colchicum—SMELLS of all kinds, gas or vomits from sight, mention or smell of FOOD. Worse from smells of meats, eggs, fish. Food taste bad. PREGNANCY. Coughing causes vomiting. Usually associated with gout.

Ipecac—PERSISTENT nausea with a clean tongue. Coughing causes nausea and vomiting. One of the top remedies for PREGNANCY and labor, with anxiety, smells, headaches, from coughs or fevers. Foods cause nausea, especially sweets, rich foods, and ice cream.

NERVE PAIN (NEURALGIA)

Nerve pains are generally tingling, burning, or numbing. These pains can be in one spot, or radiate to different parts of the body. It can be in almost any part of the body. Nerve pain is common in neuropathy of the feet, or trigeminal neuralgia in the face. Causation can be viruses that invade the nervous system for certain diseases or conditions. It may be a physical injury or problem like sciatica—shooting nerve pains down the legs. Western drugs offer a little help, and there are only a few: some cause cognitive decline and others offer severe side effects. They do not address underlying causes. Homeopathy is effective for nerve pain.

Nerve Pain Story

Many people seek help with their nerve pain, such as sciatica. It is common to take a homeopathic remedy that takes minutes to supply relief. Hypericum 30C, taken two pellets three times a day, is very effective most of the time. The best remedy is the one with the best symptom match.

Nerve Pain (Neuralgia) Essential Remedies

Aconite—nerve pains often caused by a cold dry wind, or a virus, or even from fright. Pains are TINGLING, COLD, NUMBING. Hot hands, cold feet. Despair from pains, intolerable, drives them crazy.

Arsenicum album—nerve pains are burning, but better from heat. Also, restlessness worse 10 P.M. to 2 A.M. Health fears, germs, death. Perfectionist.

Belladonna—pains are THROBBING, SHARP, come and go quickly, cutting, shooting with severe neuralgia. Can also be with delirium. Sensitive to light and noises.

Colocynthis—nerve pains are cutting, pinching, boring, afterwards followed by numbness, better from pressure on the large nerves. Facial, sciatic, spinal nerves. It has cramping, tearing pains, cutting, twisting, twitching, SHORTENING OF MUSCLES.

Hypericum—wound remedy, pinched nerves of the lower back, sacrum, coccyx (tailbone), spinal concussion, tenderness, pressure over sacrum (tailbone area). Screaming pains. Can be from surgery. RADIATING PAIN UP AND DOWN THE SPINE.

Ignatia—emotional causes or spinal injury. Cramps, twitching, spasm, tingling as if limbs asleep. Sciatica. Worse winter, better summer. JOINTS AS IF DISLOCATED. Hysterical pain.

Mag phos—FROM MUSCLE OVERUSE. Cramping pains better from heat. Facial nerve pain. All symptoms on the right side. Sciatica with sore feet. Stiff limbs.

Spigelia—nerve pains and heart disorders. Nerve pains with headaches, VIOLENT BURNING PAINS, mostly on the left side. Can't tolerate thinking of the pains. Fear of sharp things such as pins and needles.

NOSEBLEEDS

Nosebleeds can come on spontaneously with thin or thick, bright-red or dark-red blood. They may resolve in a few seconds or a few minutes, usually. Nosebleeds can come from injuries to the nose, an extra dry climate, or from picking the nose. Sometimes nosebleeds occur as a side effect of Western drugs such as blood thinners—check with your doctor and readjust the medication if symptoms are frequent. Homeopathy works quite quickly to stop the bleeding and when used regularly, avoids nosebleeds entirely.

Nosebleed Story
Sometimes when I suspect a Phosphorus personality especially in a child, they have frequent nosebleeds with bright-red blood. It can happen any time and can ruin clothes and bed sheets.

Nosebleed Essential Remedies

Agaricus—nosebleeds in the ELDERLY, dark blood. Incoherent. After alcoholism. Over talkative.

Crotalus—for SEVERE nosebleeds or hemorrhages when Phosphorus or Ferrum phos fail. Nose bleeds from septic disease. Blood is stringy, black, with flushing face, fainting or vertigo. Tip of nose cold, swollen, red and blue.

Ferrum phos—nosebleeds often associated with ANEMIA. Second remedy to try—very universal. Bright red blood. Fainting on sight of blood.

Hamamelis—slow-flow bleeding. NOSEBLEEDS PASSIVE, watery blood flow. Often in old men. Nosebleeds make most symptoms better. Dark blood.

Lachesis—rambling and over-talkative, jealous person. BLOWING THE NOSE, thick black blood. Nose bleeds with lack of menstrual periods. Often in female alcoholics.

Phosphorus—#1 remedy for nose bleeds. Frequent nosebleeds, especially in children. Bright red blood or hemorrhage. Polyps that bleed easily. Over sensitive to smells. SENSITIVE, EXTROVERT.

Secale—dark blood that oozes in broken down, scrawny old people. Also severe alcoholics or young women that also have severe menstruation. Nosebleed from the slightest touch. Worse mornings. Stringy blood. Clotted, coagulated. SUSPICIOUS, ELDERLY.

OBESITY

Nobody makes up their mind to become obese. Weight can come on in a matter of months, or take years to accumulate. Symptoms of obesity are weight gain (gradually or quickly) to the point where the person's health, mobility, and self-esteem are affected. Causation of obesity comes from overconsumption of calories and lack of exercise. The underlying cause are many, including polycystic ovarian syndrome, a hormonal issue. There are often medical reasons such as low thyroid functioning. Injuries with lack of mobility can contribute as well. Digging deeper, there may be self-esteem issues from childhood, from sexual or emotional abuse issues. Other emotional issues or causes can be the compensational eating from stress, love loss, grieving. Menopause is also a factor for many women. Western drugs may address depression (see also Grief or Depression), or even weight-loss drugs that have severe side effects. In all of this complexity, homeopathy can often address underlying issues with the correctly matched remedy. If experiencing digestive issues, *see* Gas or Bloating.

Obesity Story
Many women come to see me complaining that they can't lose the fat accompanying the last childbirth. After further details were collected, I learned that they also lost their emotional connection to family, and were doing activities out of duty. With obesity, sex with their partner feels like a duty or they become resentful and refuse. Sepia often brings them back to a loving connection with family and partner, they lose that isolation and become physically active, and lose the weight.

Obesity Essential Remedies

Aurum met—obesity with grief and depression with FINANCIAL LOSS, can have silent suicidal thoughts or actions. Feels like they have failed and then eat to compensate.

Calc carb—OBESITY AFTER PREGNANCY. Young people. Robust stout people. HOMEBODIES. Weak ankles. Can be in children. Menopause, with uterine complaints.

Capsicum—obesity in those who are HOMESICK, and sentimental. Burning pains. Elderly. Often have acne rosacea.

Ferrum met—obesity, when anemia may cause them to eat for energy, which doesn't work. Menstrual complaints. NOISE SENSITIVE.

Graphites—obesity in menopause with uterine complaints. Person with eczema especially yellow discharges behind the ears. Keloid (raised) scars. LOW SEX DRIVE.

Kali bich—IMPATIENT person with obesity. Thick yellow green mucus. Obesity in children. Alcoholism (mostly beer).

Kali carb—obesity with a RIGID PERSONALITY. RESPIRATORY PROBLEMS. Elderly. After pregnancy with uterine complaints. These are the rule keepers, but compensate with eating.

Sepia—obesity after pregnancy. As a result of HORMONAL IMBALANCES from childbirth, hormonal complaint such as uterine problems and menopause. Complains they can't lose the fat accumulated during pregnancy of their last child. Disconnects with family emotionally, wants to be alone and eats to compensate.

PALPITATIONS

Palpitations happen when the heartbeat is irregular, or, too fast or too slow. Sometimes there is no perceptible symptom. Other times, one can feel an irregularity in the chest and heart area, or can even feel the heartbeat through the chest. Here we are dealing with a condition referred to as a "nervous heart." For some people, they manifest increased or irregular heartbeats due to stressful conditions. If you have some of the symptoms, call your doctor and find out if they indicate a more serious problem. It is best to determine if it is not something more serious. A poor diet, stress, love loss, death in the family, many other things can cause this condition. It may also cause weakness or faintness. Western drugs for stress have many side effects and toxicity. Homeopathy offers help dealing with stress and then the heart may normalize.

Palpitation Story

A patient came to see me after going to a doctor. She had heart palpitations that were not linked to heart disease. She was prescribed Western drugs for anxiety, but wanted another, safer solution. Upon talking with her, I found she was a perfectionist and worried about her own health and that of her loved ones. She was convinced she had heart disease and was beginning to die. I suggested the remedy Arsenicum album. Within a few days she calmed down, the palpitations stopped, and was not worried that she would die anymore.

Palpitations Essential Remedies

Arsenicum album—the perfectionist. WORRIES about their own and their loved one's health. Palpitations are worse from excitement, physical activities, going up stairs, upon waking, with having a stool. Worse 10 P.M. to 2 A.M. Audible heartbeats.

Calc carb—workaholic. Obesity with weak ankles. Palpitations are WORSE GOING UP STAIRS, coughing, eating, evenings, and physical activity. Palpitations are audible.

Nat Mur—introvert from grief. Emotional issues such as EXCITEMENT, fear, humiliation, hysteria, and noise. Other symptoms are from going up stairs, chills, after eating, evenings, menstruation, pregnancy, waking.

Phosphoric acid—nervous physical and mental EXHAUSTION. Worse going up stairs, physical or mental work, sweating, sexual excitement. Also in children, from growing too fast.

Phosphorus—sensitive, empathetic people. Worse going up stairs, physical activity, sweating. Often from EMOTIONAL ISSUES, excitement, stress, fears, and masturbation. Also in children growing too fast.

Pulsatilla—CHANGEABLE SYMPTOMS. Weeping and whiny, needs open air. Worse evenings, mornings, going up stairs, excitement, physical activities, humiliation, joy, talking. Palpitations can also be audible and visible through the chest. Other causes: digestion of fats, coughs, after dinner.

Spigelia—heart and nerve pain. They can have headaches or migraines, palpitations often audible and visible, and come from physical activity, digestive. The heart can feel as if it stopped. They can sense it when holding breath, breathing deep, or STOOPING.

PMS

PMS symptoms include: irritability, tension, anxiety, mood swings, depression, sex drive changes, crying, bloating, pain, cramping, excessive bleeding, skin issues, and breast tenderness. Science has broken this condition down to several subcategories, but the above symptoms usually fit. Causations can be many. Often the biggest culprits are stress, hormonal changes or imbalances caused by global pollution or food chemicals, medications, and chemical birth control. Western drugs are used, such as anti-anxiety, antidepressants, as well as hormone treatment. These drugs don't address underlying weaknesses and have side effects and toxicity. Bioidentical hormones may help some symptoms but don't help the body to correct its own imbalances. Homeopathy can help correct the underlying issues if the remedy patterns match well with symptoms. The remedies can also work through hormone and drug treatment, allowing the doctor to wean the patient off some of their medications. If having other problems with menstruation, *see* Menstrual Issues.

PMS Story

Unfortunately, most women experience some or most PMS symptoms at one time or another during their childbearing years. A woman came to me declaring that she was having emotional PMS symptoms with crying, sighing, and a lump in her throat. She complained of not being able to take a satisfying deep breath. This happened a few days before her period, and continued through her period. She took the Ignatia, and within a few days most of the symptoms left and the PMS became less often in subsequent months, much to the joy of her family.

PMS Symptom/Remedy Chart

Emotional symptoms	Headaches	Breast tenderness	Uterine cramps	Profuse bleeding	Lack of period
Lachesis-nervous, irritable, jealous	Nat Mur—thousand hammers	Lac Caninum—swollen, congested	Colocynthis—anger, doubling over	Belladonna—with throbbing	Conium—repressed sexual desire
Nat Mur—introvert, worse consolation	Sulphur—throbbing band	Phytolacca—hard painful	Mag Phos—better heat, doubling over	Calc Carb—workaholic, obesity	Ferrum met—anemia
Pulsatilla—weepy, moody, better consolation	Lachesis—rush of blood to head	Calc carb—large swollen painful, obesity	Sabina*—dark clots, shooting pain	Ipecac—with nausea	Graphites—moody, obesity
Sepia—sad, depressed, worse consolation	Ignatia—frontal emotional caused	Conium—small withered celibate women	Sepia—bearing down, hormonal abnormalities	Phosphorus—bright red blood, sensitive	Ignatia—emotional causes
Ignatia—anxiety, crying, sighing					Pulsatilla—weepy, whiney
					Sepia—hormonal, low sex drive
					Silicea—thin cold, shy

*Not in Materia Medica. Not common.

PNEUMONIA

Pneumonia is an inflammation of the air sacs of the lungs. There are several types of pneumonia—from the slowly recognizable walking pneumonia, to the obvious type with painful cough, fatigue, high fevers and other symptoms. Pneumonia may occur for anyone, from infants to the elderly. Causes are many—mainly a poor diet that causes mucus (such as fast food, sugars), or from a damp environment. It may also occur from a lack of exercise. Western medicine often uses drugs such as antibiotics, which can help in emergency situations, but you can still use homeopathic medicines as they will help address underlying issues. *See also* Bronchitis and Cough, if applicable.

Pneumonia Story
In many consultations over the years, several children with pneumonia symptoms—including rattling mucus and congestion—have been helped by using homeopathic remedies. It is especially dangerous for infants as they can't cough up mucus. Most often, taking Antimonium tart in a 6X or 30C potency helps the mucus dissolve in seconds to minutes.

Pneumonia Essential Remedies

Antimonium tart—#1 remedy for pneumonia, where there is RATTLING MUCUS in the upper chest. Mucus is copious, thick and white. Croupy cough. Suffocation and shortness of breath. Last stages of pneumonia.

Phosphorus—#1 remedy for left-sided pneumonia, feeling worse lying on the left side. Hard to breathe. WHOLE BODY TREMBLES WITH COUGHING. Coughs up blood or rust-colored mucus. For chronic pneumonia in infants, children, and the elderly. Person is highly sensitive.

Arsenicum album– the perfectionist. Person is restless. Symptoms are worse from 10 P.M. to 2 A.M. Often have ALLERGIES, with SHORTNESS OF BREATH, wheezing, mucus is thick yellow and green, and a bitter taste or salty taste in the mouth.

Bryonia—pneumonia with SHARP PAINS, difficult breathing upon any movement. Must sit up to breathe. Mucus looks like jelly globs. Can't take deep breaths without coughing.

Carbo veg—pneumonia with shortness of breath, BURNING OF CHEST. Spasmodic cough and needs to be fanned. Feels like being asphyxiated from gas with pressure on the lungs. It often happens in the elderly.

Lobelia—pneumonia in infants and children. Hyperventilate easily, shortness of breath, panting, fear suffocation or death. CAN'T BREATHE BECAUSE OF CHEST CONSTRICTION. Feels a prickling sensation all over. Can't bear tobacco smoke.

Mercury sol—pneumonia when cough is croupy, often the right lung. Hard to breathe when coughing or sneezing, or going up stairs or walking quickly. Pneumonia with jaundice. WORSE IN CHANGES OF WEATHER. Useful in infants, children, and the elderly, where the cough is croupy.

PROSTATE

Many men over the age of fifty experience prostate enlargement or BPH. Prostate enlargement symptoms include perianal heaviness (one inch in front of anus), slow urinary flow, frequent urination especially at night, prostate enlargement, prostatitis, prostate cancer, erectile dysfunction, possible testicular problems. Causation can be from celibacy, sexual excesses, genital injuries, infections, sexual abuse, or other emotional trauma.

Prostate Story
An elderly man who had recently gotten married came to see me after being celibate for several years. He had prostatitis and impotence problems. After taking Conium Mac for a couple of weeks, most of his problems went away, and he and his bride were pleased.

Prostate Essential Remedies

Conium mac—effects from celibacy, or cancer risk to lower the PSA. Prostate cancer. Prostatitis, impotence, hard testicles.

Sabal Serulata—enlarged prostate BPH, prostatitis, prostate cancer, epididymitis, LOSS OF SEXUAL DESIRE. Dislikes sympathy.

Thuja—self-hate, prostatitis with PULSATING PAIN. Venereal warts, effects after gonorrhea. PROSTATE CANCER.

Chimiphila—enlarged prostate BPH, SENSATION AS IF SITTING ON A TENNIS BALL, prostate cancer, testicular atrophy. Urinary tract infections. Can't pass urine without feet apart.

Pulsatilla—emotional, people pleaser. Prostatitis, yellow discharges from gonorrhea suppressed by antibiotics. PULSATION SENSATION of prostate. Penis and testicular pains.

Selenium—ELDERLY AND IMPOTENT men, prostatitis or prostate cancer.

Staphysagria—effects from prior sexual abuse, or from anger or humiliation. From antibiotic SUPPRESSED GONORRHEA. Chronic urinary tract infection. Prostatitis and hemorrhoids, dwells on sex and masturbation. Testicle may atrophy.

PSORIASIS

Psoriasis is an autoimmune condition for which the original cause is not known. It generally manifests first with dry skin patches, mostly on the outsides of joints. These patches may form scab-like crusts. Occasionally it is associated with arthritis. Western drugs are used to relieve symptoms, are highly toxic, and suppress the immune system. There are emotional issues involved with psoriasis as well. Homeopathy can help strengthen the immune system and help the body to relieve symptoms.

Psoriasis

Psoriasis Story
Psoriasis is treatable with homeopathy, especially when there is a good symptom match. The progress is gradual. It usually takes several months, and generally other health concerns can improve too.

Psoriasis Essential Remedies

Arsenicum album—the perfectionist, with dry, scaly, itchy exfoliation of LARGE SCALES, burning and EXUDING LIQUID from a raw base.

Graphites—obesity, with dry rough skin that breaks easily and shows moist gluey eczema, but looks like honey, especially in the FOLDS OF THE SKIN; also tendency to thick scars.

Lycopodium—the skin can be SHRUNKEN, THICK, HARD, ulcerated with abscesses at the base of the psoriasis. Often with liver problems and arthritis. Worse from 4 to 8 P.M.

Nat mur—psoriasis with DRYNESS, introverted. Worse from grief or depression. With arthritis, joints are dry, burning, itching. The skin can also have a chapped or greasy and oily appearance.

Phytolacca—with swollen lymph nodes. It is accompanied with arthritis; skin is dry, shriveled, shrunken, itching, RED OR PURPLE BLOTCHES, or with blisters.

Sepia—hormonal imbalances, often with arthritis. Brownish melasma spots on face. Skin breaks down to SCALES WITH OFFENSIVE ODOR, hardens when scratched.

Staphysagria—psoriasis from humiliation, abuse, and chronic urinary tract infections. SCRATCHING CHANGES THE LOCATION OF THE ITCHING. Biting pains and unhealthy skin.

SCIATICA

Symptoms of sciatica include all kinds of pain that usually radiates from the lower back down the sciatic nerve. It can occur from the hip, shooting down to various parts of the leg—all the way to the feet in some cases. It can be in one leg or the other, and can switch sides. It can be debilitating causing limping, or sometimes total lack of mobility. Causation of sciatica is usually a back injury where the sciatic nerve is compressed, causing pain to shoot down the legs. Western medicine treatments include steroid shots, pain medications, and even surgery. Sometimes these treatments or drugs don't treat the underlying cause and have side effects. Homeopathy has shown, in my practice, to be very effective and act quite quickly. One has to be patient and try another remedy if the first one doesn't work. *See also* Nerve Pain.

Sciatic Story

A man came to see me with severe debilitating sciatic pain, starting from his right hip and shooting down the leg, causing him to limp. It was so severe that the doctor gave him steroid shots to no avail. I suggested Rhus Tox, and he found relief—within a few minutes his lower back pains also subsided and he now uses the remedy occasionally, as needed.

Sciatica Essential Remedies

Bryonia—sciatic with stabbing or SHARP PAINS only when you move, worse right side, mornings, sitting.

Colocynthis—PULSATING AND NUMBING PAIN hips to knees, better from stretching and lying on the painful side. Worse from heat, walking, touch, cold, noon, night, and motion.

Kali Iod—thin people, sciatica with lower back and tailbone pain. Limping, worse lying on painful side, sitting, standing. Wakes them up at night. Better from stretching. Skin crawls.

Mag phos—CRAMPING PAINS, shooting, sharp. Sciatica from overactivity. Causes tender feet. Worse right side. Better from warmth and pressure.

Rhus tox—sciatica with STIFFNESS worse from cold wet weather, better from continued motion. Lameness, from back injury. Cracking joints, tearing pains.

Tellurium—worse from touch, sciatica from BACK INJURY. HERNIATED DISCS. Worst at night and waking. Aching pains, worse lying on painful side.

SHINGLES

Shingles symptoms are red, inflamed, raised pustules, at first, that follow a nerve, commonly found in the abdominal area. They can be burning or itching. The pustules clear up but the pains may remain—usually burning at any time. It can last days, weeks, months or years. Causation of shingles is the herpes virus, which attacks the nerve branches. The pains follow the nerves. It can come on from eating a poor diet, poor sleep, and long-time stress. Someone with a long-lasting condition or disease may also be vulnerable. Western drugs such as antivirals will help the symptoms, but cause liver damage and don't help with nerve weakness. Homeopathic remedies stimulate the body to repair the nerves. The correct remedy usually works in two to seven days, maybe less.

Shingles Story
A woman came to me with painful shingle pustules on her thighs. Her doctor had prescribed an antiviral and told her she should find relief in two weeks. I recommended Ranunculus bulbosa. She used it, and in less than twenty-four hours the pain went away. Her pustules cleared up in a few more days.

Shingles Essential Remedies

Ranunculus bulbosa—useful for acute and chronic shingles with blisters that burn and itch. Worse from touch. This especially good for the RIB area.

Rhus tox—acute and chronic shingles that burn, hot needles, intense itching. Often associated with joint STIFFNESS.

Clematis—shingles in the SCALP area that are worse washing in cold water. Red burning scaly and scabby. Especially in smokers.

Iris versicolor—shingles with digestive problems, with pancreatic problems, severe itching at night.

Mercury Sol—shingles worse when TOUCHED. Burning, worse from heat of bed. RESTLESSNESS.

Mezereum—shingles with burning pains, ERUPTIONS OOZE, gluey with scabs and pus underneath. Worse at night. Chronic and post-shingles eruption pains.

Nat Mur—shingles and other types of herpes. DRY SKIN, worse in flexures (inner side of joint), chapped skin. INTROVERT, shingles worse grieving or other stress. Burning pain.

SINUSES

Sinus symptoms are mainly congestion, with or without infection or pain. Other symptoms can include mucus discharges, with or without an infection, and blood in mucus. Most mucus congestion is caused by digestive insufficiency, which causes mucus to build up in the digestive tract and spill over into the sinuses and lungs. The sinuses can be affected by wind, or exposure to cold. There may also be an infection evidenced by yellow-green mucus, or contain dried blood. Western drugs offered for sinus problems are mostly antibiotics that can give temporary relief. But these drugs don't target underlying conditions, are toxic, and negatively affect colon probiotics. Homeopathy tends to be very

Sinuses

effective and can relieve symptoms in minutes or hours. *See also* Mucus or Sore Throat, if applicable.

Sinus Story
People frequently come in for a consultation for their sinusitis. The two main remedies that work are Kali Bich when the mucus is green and thick, and Pulsatilla where there are changeable mucus conditions.

Sinus Essential Remedies

Kali bich—#1 remedy for sinus. Has YELLOW-GREEN, THICK MUCUS. Bones in head feel sore, dull, throbbing. Can have post-nasal drip.

Thuja—#2 remedy for sinus. GREEN MUCUS, mostly left frontal sinuses with postnasal drip. The head feels numb and heavy.

Hydrastis*—yellow-green mucus, often with headaches, POSTNASAL DRIP. Affects the frontal sinuses. Better dry weather, worse cold air.

Lycopodium—right-sided sinus with postnasal drip. Symptoms worse 4 to 8 P.M. Liver issues.

Mercury sol—BURNING SINUSITIS, frontal sinus, often with headaches, green mucus. Restless. Postnasal drip.

Pulsatilla– CHANGEABLE SYMPTOMS as well as changeable mucus. Better in open air.

Silicea—SENSITIVE TO COLD DRAFTS including air conditioners in the summer. Feels better wrapping up the head. Has postnasal drip. Greenish mucus. Thin, delicate people.

*Not in Materia Medica. Not common.

SLEEP PROBLEMS (INCLUDING INSOMNIA)

Having a hard time getting to sleep or staying asleep? Could be many reasons: injury, arthritis, pains of any kind including headaches, stiffness, stress, grief, overactive mind. Any of these can keep you from falling or staying asleep. It is best to ascertain what conditions or symptoms are preventing a good night sleep. Western drugs for these conditions can force people to sleep. They're often toxic, cause memory problems, and worse of all, they disrupt sleep cycles, affecting a person's mental health. Homeopathy can regulate sleep cycles by helping the body to work optimally. It does take at least 30 days to establish a healthy sleep cycle.

Sleep Story

People frequently ask about their insomnia, as it is affecting everything in their life. If the mind is too active, the remedy Coffea Cruda before bed generally helps. If there is stiffness and aching, Rhus Tox is quite effective to calm aches and pains, and good sleep follows.

Sleep Problem Essential Remedies

Arsenicum album—sleepless to 3 A.M., talks in sleep, dreams of bad things, nervous exhaustion. Restless and anxious 10 P.M. to 2 A.M. Perfectionist. WORRIES ABOUT THEIR HEALTH.

Capsicum—sleeplessness from emotions, HOMESICKNESS. Dreams of falling from heights. Burning pains, can also contribute to sleeplessness.

Coffea cruda —insomnia from EMOTIONAL CARES or EXCESSIVE CAFFEINE. Pleasant dreams. Also, may have an itching anus. Mind talks too much.

Hepar sulph—sleep problems with OVERSENSITIVITY, irritability, bad-tempered. Pain makes everything worse. Worse with drafts.

Kali ars—perfectionist, PANIC ATTACKS. Asthma worse 1 to 4 A.M. Sleeps with hand over the heart. Nightmares, vivid dreams.

Kali carb—obesity. Rule keeper. Can't sleep after 2 to 4 A.M. WAKES UP AND CAN'T GO BACK TO SLEEP. Sleep during daytime, sleepless from coughing, and before menstruation.

Nux vomica—sleepless from stimulant abuse, alcohol, addictive drugs. Caused from mental stress. Can't sleep after 3 A.M. MENTAL EXHAUSTION, sweating at night. Feels hot. Erotic dreams.

Silicea—thin, cold, shy people. Sleepy during the day, SLEEPWALKING, sleep TALKING, dreams of past events or nightmares. Unrefreshing sleep.

SORE THROAT

Sore throat symptoms include pain, redness, hard to swallow, and swelling. May also have pus in the throat, and swollen lymph nodes. There are several types of pain and constriction in sore throats. Causation can be from a strep infection, postnasal drip, or a sinus infection. Western drugs usually employ antibiotics that are toxic and don't get to the other underlying causes. Homeopathy tends to help the body reduce pain, usually in as soon as a few minutes or just a couple of days. *See also* Sinus or Flu.

Sore Throat Story
It's frequent to get calls for sore throats in my practice. The correctly matched homeopathic remedy takes just a few minutes to relieve pain and discomfort, amazingly. Belladonna is frequently used, 30C at two pellets three times a day, and can relieve pain in as little as five to ten minutes, when the sore throat has throbbing pains, and possible high fever.

Sore Throat Essential Remedies

Argentum nitricum—sore throat with panic attacks. Burning, DRYNESS, SPLINTER-LIKE PAIN, feels as if strangled. With voice loss from talking, singing, or overuse.

Belladonna—sore throats with FEARS AND DELIRIUM, throat feels constricted, throbbing pain as if something were caught in the throat. Scraping sensation. With possible high fever.

Calc carb—SWOLLEN TONSILS AND UVULA, throat worse from wet weather, talking. Sharp pains when swallowing. Salty mucus taste. From overwork. Obesity.

Ignatia—hysterical throat spasms. Sighing, crying, LUMP-IN-THROAT SENSATION. Can't swallow, with hoarseness and voice trembling.

Lachesis—Constricting throat, worse swallowing liquid. Doesn't want anything touching their throat. TALKATIVE, EXTROVERTED.

Lycopodium—Chronically enlarged tonsils, ulceration. Sharp pains. Feels worse 4 to 8 P.M., cold drinks. Better with warm drinks.

Mercury Sol—sore throat with excess SALIVA, loss of voice, tonsils enlarged. Glands enlarged. Restless, worse night. Gums may be involved.

Nitric acid—SPLINTER-LIKE PAINS. Worse singing, talking, loss of voice. Dry hacking cough. Tonsils red, swollen, ulcerated. Pessimistic.

SWEATING

As the skin releases moisture, we sweat. The sweat can be hot or cold, excessive, odorous, or mild. There may be fever, hormonal issues (during menstrual years or menopause). Sweating is the body's way to create equilibrium and regulate temperature under normal circumstances. It

Sweating

is the body's defense against bacteria, viruses. First the body increases heat to improve the immune system and hinder the bacteria or virus. Many people sweat as a result of a week nervous system, or have stress-induced perspiration. Disease can cause sweating.

Sweating Story

A young man came to see me. He was thin, cold and complained of offensive-smelling foot sweat. He took the remedy Silicea, and the offensive foot sweat went away in a couple of weeks, as his overall energy was improved.

Sweating Essential Remedies

Ant tart—profuse cold sweat that brings no relief; person feels clammy; SWEATING IS DEBILITATING. Mucus with the rattling in the chest. Also from fevers.

Calc carb—obesity. Has COLD, CLAMMY, debilitating sweat. Sour sweat; sweats after eating and more at night, which causes weakness.

China/Cinchona—weakness from excess or PROFUSE SWEATING, or other fluid loss. Anxiety. Worse from physical exertion. Can also be from a fever. Emotional oversensitivity.

Hepar sulph—sensitivity, anxiety and irritability. Profuse, COLD, CLAMMY, and debilitating sweat. Sweat is sour, with an offensive bad-smelling odor, which gives no relief.

Lycopodium—anxiety and fears cause sweating. Sweating is cold, clammy, sour with bad-smelling odor. It is PROFUSE, DEBILITATING, worse at night.

Nat mur—ANXIETY FROM GRIEF. Introverted. Sweat is clammy, cold, worse from eating, exertion, and is debilitating. Craves salt.

Nux vomica—anxiety and irritability. From ALCOHOL, DRUGS OR STIMULANTS. Sweat is sour with offensive odor, cold or hot, and is debilitating. Sweating brings no relief. Digestive problems.

Phosphorus—SWEATING FROM ANXIETY, fright, or menstruation. Sweat is cold, clammy, debilitating, bad smelling odor. Worse from exertion, and eating. Sweating causes no relief.

Sepia—HORMONAL CAUSES FROM MENSTRUATION, anxiety and fright of strangers. Anxiety around strangers and fright. Sweat is profuse, sour and bad smelling. Sweat gives no relief. Debilitating, worse at night, with eating, exertion.

Silicea—sweat from fright and anxiousness. The SWEAT IS SOUR, PROFUSE, weakening, from exertion; odor is bad smelling, especially on the FEET. Thin, cold, delicate people.

TEETHING

In babies and children, cutting their first set of teeth causes pain, and sometimes diarrhea. Crying, swollen tonsils, irritability, and even canker sores in the mouth, accompany the main symptoms. Causation is the teeth pushing through the gums, which creates the above symptoms.

Teething Story
I frequently have mothers calling me about their children who are experiencing irritability, pain and diarrhea while teething. I will usually recommend the remedies Chamomilla and Belladonna taken together, and taken every few hours. Many mothers report that the baby's symptoms are mostly diminished usually in a day or less.

Teething Essential Remedies

Aconite—gums are HOT, SWOLLEN and inflamed. Green stools.

Arsenicum album—feels better from warmth. Symptoms worse from 10 P.M. to 2 A.M. GUMS AND TEETH ARE COVERED IN SLIME.

Belladonna—anger, gums red and hot, swollen. Throbbing pains with a red-hot face. May have convulsions with high fevers, and can grind teeth.

Borax—CANKER SORES ON THE TONGUE, mouth hot and sensitive purse. Nursing causes crying.

Calc carb—FAT BABIES, SMELL SOUR. Milk disagrees, can have convulsions. With swollen tonsils.

Calc phos—DELAYED TEETHING, has colic after feeding, child hard to please. Growing pains, diarrhea.

Chamomilla—#1 remedy for teething. WANTS TO BE HELD BUT IS DISSATISFIED, angry. Can have convulsions. Green, spinach-like diarrhea. Colic, insomnia.

Mercury sol—teething with EXCESSIVE SALIVA; thick, yellow mucus, gums are swollen and spongy, swollen glands. Worse in change of temperature or weather. Can have chronic earaches.

Silicea—delayed teething. Thin, shy, delicate, cold and weak children.

TOOTHACHES

Toothache symptoms include pain, aching, throbbing, sharp pains, possible spongy gums, and infections. Pain may be affected by hot or cold temperature, contact, or movement. The main cause of toothache is poor nutrition, or excess sugar consumption, which leaches calcium. Calcium deficiency is the number one reason for toothaches. It can also come from tooth injuries, including nerve damage. *See also* Gums, if applicable.

Toothaches Story
Before they can get to see their dentist, clients consult me frequently for advice on their toothaches. I generally recommend liquid calcium

and the homeopathic Calc Phos 6x as a cell salt, taken several times a day. It will usually calm toothaches within a few days. Then I use a more specific remedy for the pain of the toothache.

Toothache Essential Remedies

Aconite—SENSITIVE TO COLD AND DRY WINDS, especially cold in thenhealthy teeth. Throbbing and grinding. Causation is from fright or exposure to cold dry winds.

Belladonna—intolerable THROBBING PAIN, better from biting down. Face is red, hot and throbbing. Usually right-sided with right cheek red and hot. Accompanied by headaches, grinding teeth and swollen gums. Worse in cold air and from draft.

Bryonia—toothaches when coughing, brushing teeth, smoking, chewing tobacco, and at 3 A.M. Nerve pain in tooth from cold air. TEETH FEEL TOO LONG. Better from cold water. Pains sharp especially upon movement, more on the right side of the mouth.

Chamomilla—worse when entering a warm room. Bad breath. BETTER DRINKING COFFEE. Thirsty for hot drinks. Wants instant relief of suffering, demanding. One of the cheeks is red. Worse 9 P.M. to midnight.

China/Cinchona—TEETH LOOSE, painful, gums swollen. Toothache better from biting down, with heat and from sweating, nursing. Pressure, pain sensation with throbbing and better from warmth. Worse chewing, cold air, and draft.

Coffea cruda—TOOTHACHES WITH ICE WATER in the mouth. Worse from any emotional excitement. Intolerable pain with restlessness, anxiety, crying. Frequently in children, worse chewing.

Mercury sol—loose teeth, tender, FEEL TOO LONG. Roots of teeth inflamed, ulcerate and fall out. Often at night, with chills, excessive saliva. Worse from heat or cold and at night. Teeth can be hollow, black, decayed. Spongy gums. Shooting pains.

Staphysagria—TEETH OFTEN GREY OR BLACK, crumbling. Tearing pain, worse with any food in decayed teeth. Pain into roots worse during menstruation and pregnancy, and from cold. Teeth and gums painful in teething in children.

TRAVEL SICKNESS

Travel sickness is also called "motion sickness," "seasickness," or "morning sickness." It happens when any type of motion causes vertigo or dizziness, nausea, vomiting, or generally a feeling of unwellness while in a moving vehicle, or moving physically. Some people are just prone to travel sickness. It is worse from alcohol and lack of sleep. Western drugs tend to offer antihistamines to help symptoms. The side effect is cognitive or mental decline while you are using it. *See also* Nausea and Vomiting.

Travel Sickness Story
Hoping to avoid the use of pharmaceutical drugs, customers ask my advice for travel sickness relief. Generally, I recommend Cocculus as it can help almost immediately for most people. If it doesn't, we look to the following remedies.

Travel Sickness Essential Remedies

Cocculus indicus—traveling causes migraines. #1 remedy for travel sickness. Better sitting, lying quietly, worse from motion, kneeling, walking, touch, pain, sun, night. VERTIGO WITH NAUSEA and vomiting. Heart palpitations. Motion sickness from loss of sleep. Feels faint, even intoxicated.

Petroleum—ravenous hunger, nausea, green vomiting, seasickness. NAUSEA IN PREGNANCY better from stooping (leaning over). Worse promotion: dampness, cold weather, winter, weather change, and touch. Better from warmth, dryness, head held high.

Tabaccum—nausea, giddiness, SEVERE SINKING-STOMACH SENSATION. Vomiting, cold sweating. Seasickness. Migraine with nausea, vertigo. Fluttering, shocks in the stomach. Sinking feeling in the bottom of the stomach. Pregnancy, worse morning.

Conium—headache with nausea and vomiting of mucus. Vertigo lying down, turning over in bed. Worst turning head, eyes, shaking head, noises, conversation.

Nux vomica—problems of travel sickness made worse from drugs or stimulants. Feels bloated, must loosen belt. Sour taste and nausea in the morning. Hiccups from overeating. Nausea and vomiting, seasickness.

TREMORS

These tremor symptoms parallel non-Parkinson's pill-rolling movements—involuntary movements that cause a person's muscles not to function normally. The movements are generally random and non-uniform. Causation is some sort of nervous system failure to control muscle movement. It can come from extreme stress conditions and/or sleep deprivation. A poor diet may contribute. This condition may be an inherited weakness called a "familial tremor." Bodily toxicity can also play a part.

Tremors Story
I have dealt with non-Parkinson's familial tremors several times. One client was a man who applied gold leaf for a living, but his hands couldn't do the fine details anymore. I suggested Zinc Met 30C, three times a day. In a few days, he was back to work. He used the remedy for three months, and the effects became permanent.

Tremors Essential Remedies

Agaricus—limbs are TREMBLING AND TWITCHING, muscle soreness. Trembling on walking. Has stiffness, sensitive to the cold. Itching of toes and limbs, as if frozen. Worse cold, alcohol.

Causticum—TWISTING AND JERKING MOVEMENTS. Paralysis of single parts, unsteady muscles, contracted tendons. Joints burn. Walking unsteady, falls easily. Can have electric shocks in legs. Feels better cold damp air and weather. Symptoms worse 3 to 4 A.M. and 6 to 8 P.M.

Cuprum Met—has CONVULSIVE MOVEMENTS especially at night with jerking and clenching of thumbs in the palms of the hands. Twitching as well as convulsions.

Nux vomica—has liver weakness, alcohol and stimulant abuse. Digestive problems. Symptoms worse 3 A.M. CONVULSIVE WALKING, cramps with shocks, loss of strength, trembling and shooting pain.

Zinc Met—FEET IN CONTINUED MOTION and restless. Weakness, trembling, twitching, can't stop motion of different muscles. Walks with spasms. Soles of feet sensitive. Often has large varicose veins.

URINARY TRACT INFECTIONS (UTI)

Symptoms of urinary tract infections include pain, stinging, burning, urgency to urinate, increased frequency, discoloration, change in urine odor, leaking, dribbling urine. Causes can be many—from past emotional or sexual abuse, or bacterial contamination from unsanitary conditions such as personal hygiene (sexual partner affected too). Western drugs only offer antibiotics with their toxicity, ruining our microbiome. Homeopathy can help the body to resolve underlying conditions and provide relief in hours to a couple of days. *See also* Incontinence, if applicable.

Urinary Tract Infection Story

A woman, in her late thirties, consulted with me for recur recurring UTIs, especially after intercourse. She said that she had to take antibiotics before each time she had sex with her partner. In our consultation, she also revealed she had been sexually abused as a child. I suggested Staphysagria, and within two weeks she was able to have sex without using antibiotics, and after a month the UTIs never returned.

Urinary Tract Infections Essential Remedies

Aconite—SHARP AND STINGING PAINS in the kidney region. The urine is scanty, red, hot and painful. Worse from fright, or cold dry winds.

Argentum nit—sharp, burning, ITCHING PAIN. Worse touching kidney and urethra areas. Craves sugar, which makes it worse.

Belladonna—THROBBING, BURNING, STINGING PAINS. Profuse, frequent urination that is dark, cloudy, thick. Sudden onset, involuntary urination.

Cantharis—#1 remedy for urinary tract infections. Stinging, smarting, burning, biting, cutting. There is also DROP BY DROP DRIBBLE.

Causticum—from HOLDING URINE TOO LONG in labor, or from surgery. Urethra burns after sex. The urine dribbles, passes slowly, cloudy. Incontinence and involuntary passing of urine.

Mercury corrosive—hot burning frequent urination and kidney inflammation. URINE HAS A GREENISH DISCHARGE. Restless especially at night. Painful, drop by drop, and sweats afterward.

Nux vomica—urine dribbles in OLD MEN WITH PROSTATE PROBLEMS. Ineffectual urging to urinate, with mucus. Worse from stimulants and drug abuse.

Pulsatilla—pain with urging to urinate when lying on back. CRAMPING AFTER URINATION, bleeding after urination. Incontinence. Cries easily.

Staphysagria—cause is sexual abuse, rape. Chronic UTIs, ESPECIALLY AFTER SEX. Also, prostate problems. Pain after lithotripsy or kidney stones.

Terebinthina—urine is ODOR OF VIOLETS. Burning and drawing pains along the urethra or ureters. Radiating pain, bladder to naval, urine is bloody, thick and muddy.

VARICOSE VEINS

Veins in the legs can be painful from the thighs down. Either leg, or both, can be affected from old age, injury, or pregnancy. Pains can be sharp, burning, or throbbing. It can cause weakness. When worst they can bleed. Veins can be also large and unsightly. Causation is poor circulation from inherited family traits, made worse by a poor diet, injuries, obesity, pregnancy, or lack of activity. Western medicine recommends surgery. All surgeries require risk and maybe a temporary fix if the underlying issue is not addressed. Many people are interested in non-surgical solutions to varicose veins and homeopathy can address pain and inflammation and sometimes the appearance.

Varicose Vein Story
A woman consulted with me complaining of varicose vein pain, almost as soon as she became pregnant. It was especially painful on her labia—she was an in agony walking and moving around. Hamamelis took care of the pain, almost immediately. And, after using it for a few more weeks, she was fine throughout the rest of her pregnancy.

Varicose Veins Essential Remedies

Arnica—varicose veins FROM INJURIES. Sore, bruised, lameness. Can use with phlebitis or varicose ulcers. Use in pregnancy with symptoms.

Calcarea fluorica—for hard veins, worse from warmth, with dermatitis, varicosities, LEG ULCERS. Also feels restless.

Carbo veg—blue tissues, weak legs, cold from the knees down in lower legs, legs feel asleep. Venous stasis, ULCERATION. Pregnancy with gas and bloating.

Fluoric acid—LOWER LEGS, left leg, sensitive, feeble legs, legs go to sleep. Useful in pregnancy.

Hamamelis—lower legs, THIGHS PAINFUL, sensitive. Inflamed veins to varicose ulcers, hemorrhoids, sore nipples, pregnancy varicose labia.

Lycopodium—lower legs, more right-sided and painful, ulceration, BLOOD CLOTS, pregnancy.

Pulsatilla—thighs, lower legs. Worse with warmth. LEGS FEEL HEAVY AND COLD. Varicose veins are sensitive, swollen, pelvic pulsating. There is venous stasis, varicose ulcers. Pregnancy with crying, indecision.

Zinc met—thighs, lower legs inflamed, cramping, RESTLESS LEGS, trembling, twitching, lameness, formication (sensation of bugs crawling under skin). Nerve weakness, pregnancy, seizures.

VISION ISSUES

Vision is impaired in some way to hamper normal sight. This could be poor night vision, blurriness, dimness, colors altered, partial vision, central or peripheral vision disturbances. Chinese medicine claims that vision problems are linked to the liver and its health. Other causations are injuries to the retina, chemical poisoning, and Western pharmaceutical drugs. *See also* Macular Degeneration, if applicable.

Vision Story
I have had several cases of people with central vision loss. Carboneum sulph has been remarkable in partially, or fully, restoring the central vision problem over days to weeks.

Vision Essential Remedies

Agaricus—fearful. Eyes weak, spasm, TWITCHING EYELIDS, EYEBALLS. Sensitive to light, pupils dilated. Causation—alcoholism. Overconfident.

Allium cepa—nerve pains from allergies. Causation from wind or surgical. Like cutting a red onion, eyes burn, red, smart, lots of bland tears, EYES LIGHT SENSITIVE. Eyelids burn. Torn sensation. Vision—letters seem smaller.

Carboneum sulph—LOSS OF CENTRAL VISION. Atrophy of retina, myopia. Reading causes tears. Eyelids heavy and sore.

Euphrasia (eyebright herb)—allergies, as if SAND IN EYES. Watery eyes in allergies. Eyes water all the time. Yellow mucus. Profuse, hot, burning tears. Conjunctivitis with mucus. Corneal blisters. Sensitive to light. Burning and swelling of eyelids. Injuries cause cataracts.

Gelsemium—panic attacks. DROOPY EYELIDS, eyes twitching. Sore when moving eyes, glaucoma, can't keep eyes open. Retinitis, detached retina. One pupil dilated the other contracted. Double vision.

Nitric acid—HEALTH FEARS. Sharp stitching pains and eyes. Inflammation of the iris, paralysis of the upper eyelid.

Phosphorus—#1 remedy for most vision and retinal issues. RETINAL ATROPHY, bleeding, degeneration, yellow eyes. Sensitive to light, feels large (sensation like being swollen), sand in left eye, better rubbing. Glaucoma, cataracts. Caused by fears, such as electrocution. Intuitive, ungrounded.

Sulphuric acid—#1 remedy for blood in the eyes. Causation— INJURIES OR SURGERIES. Blood in eyes, painful conjunctiva. Eyes burn, smart, lots of tears especially when reading. Feels hurried.

Nat sulph—HEAD INJURIES cause eye problems or blindness. Eye problems, seizures, depression. From head injury—sensitive to light, hot, itching worse reading, weak eyes, confused sight, sparks. Conjunctivitis, yellow or green pus.

WARTS

Warts are fleshy growths that can emerge on almost any part of the body, except the eyeballs. They are not normally painful, but can be. They have different shapes and are unsightly. Warts are generally abnormal non-cancerous growths caused by viruses of unknown origin. Western medicine cuts or burns the war topically, and then they grow back. The underlying cause is not addressed. Homeopathy is quite efficient.

Warts Story
I met with a woman who had 28 fleshy warts on her hands. I suggested the remedy Thuja. She used Thuja 30C, two pellets once a day. In 30 days they were gone without a trace! When the symptoms match, warts generally take 30 to 60 days to go away.

Warts

Warts Essential Remedies

Antimonium crud—fungus, warts. Smooth warts. #1 remedy for
PLANTAR WARTS. Horny warts on hands, soles of feet. Digestive
issues. Tender feet. #3 remedy for warts.

Calc carb—warts in obese people. The warts are small and painful,
soft bleeding, fleshy or hard, most JAGGED, itching, or moist.

Causticum—large seed warts, EASILY BLEEDING. Jagged ulceration. Mostly on fingertips, nose, eyelids, or eyebrows, under fingernails, and on the face. #2 remedy for warts.

Dulcamara—warts that are SMOOTH, FLAT or fleshy in groups of
small or large size. Facial, hand, finger warts.

Nitric acid—warts with SPLINTER-LIKE PAINS. Large and jagged, soft, burning, itching, moist, mostly small but painful warts.
Negative emotions.

Thuja—#1 remedy for warts. Has almost all of the above symptoms,
pains, sizes. FINDS THEIR WARTS DISGUSTING.

CHAPTER 3

Materia Medica
Remedy Guide with
Keynotes And Symptoms

Let's learn the remedies and their symptom pictures. As you come to understand the KEYNOTES of a few remedies, when you are actually experiencing those symptoms and need it, the right remedy will come to mind. It will become like second nature.

As talked about in Chapter 1, Dr. Hahnemann and his staff were able to record the symptoms of each patient in a homeopathic "proving." These symptoms were compiled into a Materia Medica, or Remedy Guide, which is a compilation of the symptoms of hundreds of homeopathic medicines that have been proven (and used) for up to 200 years, and more. These remedies will be found in alphabetical order and contain different headings that separate the symptoms into categories (Mind symptoms, Body symptoms, Clinical uses, etc.).

You may have noticed while looking through the previous chapter, there were homeopathic remedies that were utilized for many conditions, i.e., Arsenicum, Mercury Sol, or Sepia, to name a few. These are called "polychrests," defined as "a drug medicine of value, as a remedy in several diseases." These are the top, most used, homeopathic remedies, which treat 70 percent to 90 percent of health conditions. I use these remedies much of the time, and so will you. Polychrests comprise 50 to 60 homeopathic remedies, yet everyone who studies homeopathy seriously has their own opinion as to how many there really are.

In this Materia Medica or Remedy Guide, each remedy is listed in alphabetical order, with its Latin name and the material or substance from which it is made. One of the most important features of each remedy is KEYNOTES, which will help you distinguish the remedy that fits your symptoms the closest. Then, sometimes mental symptoms, personalities, or gender play a role, or the time of day you are having symptoms (under Modalities). Remember, you don't have to have all the symptoms of a remedy in order for it to work well, it doesn't need to be an exact match. The following list comprises the categories or headings I find most helpful when choosing a remedy:

- **KEYNOTES.** The most important symptoms of the remedy; they will lead you to success the fastest. It is the summary of the remedy. These keynotes are based on symptoms that differentiate the remedy from others for a precise match. Among the KEYNOTES you will find:

  - **Physical symptoms** are very important to get a good match, but nobody has all the symptoms. Your symptoms should be in there, but you won't have all of them, nor should you. If you have mental symptoms only, the physical symptoms may not be as helpful.

  - **Mental symptoms** can be very significant. You don't have to have them all, but a general pattern. Mental symptoms can range in intensity from slight, to irritation, to anxiety, to hallucinations. Homeopathy can cover the whole spectrum.

- **MODALITIES (Worse or Better)** help finetune the symptom match. Look at the better or worse symptoms that apply to your case. Times when these problems happen may be important but are not always relevant.

- **ASSOCIATED**
  - **Sides** often indicate where the majority of the symptoms occur. If everything else fits but the side doesn't, then ignore the side.
  - **Organs** are indicative, and generally helpful.
  - **Gender** can be valuable as well, but occasionally will not fit your symptom picture. Whether male or female, you can have masculine or feminine qualities.
  - **Personalities** may indicate a person's profession or their common mental state.
  - **Causations** can be valuable, recognizing when the ailment came on, and why.
  - **Common Health Issues** indicate what the remedy has treated historically but is not exclusive to everything the remedy can do. I have used a remedy for specific conditions and many times my client will report that other health problems have gone away.

USE OF UPPER CASE:

As noted in previous chapters, UPPER CASE indicates a "defining action," that is, a primary symptom.

ACONITE
Aconitum Napellus (Monkshood)

KEYNOTES
Effects from FRIGHT, SHOCK, worse from cold wind.

SYMPTOMS
Physical symptoms—colds and flu with sudden onset, illness that starts at NOON. Fever, restlessness, and thirsty with red swollen face. Eyes, pupils contracted. Vertigo with nausea. Burning thirst. Hyperventilating in a warm room. Pneumonia in children. Raised blood pressure. Excessive bleeding of bright red blood.

Mental/Emotional symptoms—NWS (never well since) FRIGHT or MEMORY OF FRIGHT. Aversion to being touched, restless, sensitive to noise or music. Bites fingernails. Despair and rage with PAIN, groans, shrieks. Openminded. Fears future and crowds. Panic attacks.

MODALITIES
Worse—night, from fright or shock, cold dry winds, noise or music, light, teething in children, tobacco smoke, and rising from bed. Better—in open air, rest, warm sweating. Times—worse at night.

ASSOCIATED
Sides—right.
Organs—brain, chest, heart, nerves, joints.
Gender—masculine or feminine.
Personalities—agriculture, sports, strong body.
Causation—frights and cold winds.
Common Health Issues—chills, colds and flu, croup in children, fears, fevers, FRIGHTS, heart attack, heart palpitations, nightmares, panic attacks.

AESCULUS HIPP
Aesculus Hippocastanum (Horse Chestnut)

KEYNOTES
HIPS, HEMORRHOIDS, LOWER BACK, VARICOSE VEINS

SYMPTOMS
Physical symptoms—mucus membranes dry, swollen, burning sensation, raw; mucus is thin, watery, burning. Fatigue, chilliness. Hhemorrhoids, liver congestion. Skin coloration, dark red or purple. Pain in sacroiliac joint. Hip pains with degeneration, worse walking or stooping. Weak veins, enlarged.

Mental/Emotional symptoms—dullness, confusion on waking, irritable, sensation of impending death. Depressed, irritable.

MODALITIES
Worse—waking, stool, urination, walking, sleep, rest, stooping, warm room. Better—cool, continued motion, air, water, summer, bleeding hemorrhoids (relieves), kneeling. Times—worse mornings, waking, sleep.

ASSOCIATED
Sides—right.

Organs—mucus membranes, spine, abdomen, veins, rectum.

Gender—masculine or feminine.

Personalities—not important.

Causations—hemorrhoids, menopause, varicose veins.

Common Health Issues—arthritis, back ache, glandular swelling, hemorrhoids, hip joints, sacroiliac pain, varicose veins.

AGARICUS
Agaricus Muscarius (Aminita Mushroom)

KEYNOTES
Twitching, nervousness, health anxiety, excitement or ecstasy.

SYMPTOMS
Physical symptoms—rolls their head, "magical look" in eyes, other eye issues (swing like pendulum, eyes crossed), cracked lower lip (Nat Mur), involuntary yawning and/or laughter, grimacing, jerking, twitching, tics, epilepsy, physical awkwardness.

Mental/Emotional symptoms—exaggerated emotions, mental excitement, ecstasy, anxious, talkative (going from subject to subject) (Lachesis), embracing, kisses hands of others, laughs loudly. Fearlessness alternating with lots of fears of cancer, dying, ghosts, graveyards. Self-pity.

MODALITIES
Worse—COLD, stormy weather, mental effort, pressure, touch, motion, menstruation, thunderstorms. Better—evenings, gentle motion. Times—better mornings.

ASSOCIATED
Sides—right.
Organs—spinal cord, nervous system.
Gender—masculine or feminine.
Personalities—end-of-life caretakers, undertakers.
Causation—frostbite, over excitement, alcoholism.
Common Health Issues—alcoholism, frostbite, tics, twitching.

ALLIUM
Allium Cepa (Red Onion)

KEYNOTES
Irritating discharges, burning, mucus, bland tears.

SYMPTOMS
Physical symptoms—mucus constitutions, bland tears, RAW—especially nose, with irritating, watery discharges. Sinusitis with mucus and swelling. Allergies with irritating discharges and bland tears. Yellow teeth.

Mental/Emotional symptoms—not important

MODALITIES
Worse—WARMTH, DAMPNESS, evenings. Better—COOL, open air, motion. Times—worse 2 A.M., mornings.

ASSOCIATED
Sides—left.

Organs—mucus membranes, lymphatics.

Gender—masculine or feminine.

Personalities—singers with mucus conditions.

Causations—cold damp weather.

Common Health Issues—allergies, colds, mucus conditions, sneezing.

ALUMINA
Alumina (Oxide of Aluminum)

KEYNOTES
DRY, severe CONSTIPATION, OLD, EMACIATED

SYMPTOMS
Physical symptoms—Head-hair loss, dandruff. Eyes, strabismus. Cracks in tip of nose. Dryness. CONSTIPATION, weakened conditions with constipation—even soft stools badly passed with straining. Stool is hard, dry, sheep dung-like. Drags left foot. Lax ligaments and joints, weak nerves. Sedentary, sluggish with vague symptoms. Any chronic ailment. Generally looks old, wrinkled. Girls in puberty, or weak children. All symptoms worse on waking.

Mental/Emotional symptoms—confused, obstinate, dull, makes mistakes, can't be hurried. Fears of pointy objects, slowed thought, conscience feels guilty, confusion of identity. Sighing, no smiling.

MODALITIES
Worse—waking, warmth, food sensitivities, cold, winter, new or full moons. Better—everything moderate (temperature, food, etc.), wet weather. Times—better in evenings.

ASSOCIATED
Sides—right.

Organs—spine, mucus membranes, skin, rectum.

Gender—masculine or feminine.

Personalities—not important.

Causation—disappointments, overexertion.

Common Health Issues—ALS (amyotrophic lateral sclerosis), CONSTIPATION (severe), emaciation, Multiple Sclerosis.

ANTIMONIUM CRUD
Antimonium Crudum (Sulphide of Antimony)

KEYNOTES
SKIN—calluses—hard brittle, worse cold damp

SYMPTOMS
Physical symptoms—tongue coated white, thick. Glutton or obese. Chronic indigestion. Wants large amounts of food and acid or sour foods. Split or brittle nails. Nail fungus. Calluses on feet or toes or horny, split skin. Calluses on soles of feet. Impetigo. Warts on soles of the feet.

Mental/Emotional symptoms—romantic person, sentimental, moonlight. Idealistic, with harsh voice, talks in rhymes. Anger when touched, and irritable. Children don't like to be looked at.

MODALITIES
Worse—cold, damp, water, overeating, heat and sun, in temperature extremes. Better—warm bath, rest, open air, vomiting. Times—worse in evening, night, and moonlight.

ASSOCIATED
Sides—left.

Organs—digestive tract, skin.

Gender—masculine or feminine.

Personalities—cold water work.

Causation—disappointed love, sun overheating.

Common Health Issues—belching, brittleness, gout, nail fungus, impetigo, rashes, skin calluses, warts.

ANTIMONIUM TART
Antimonium tartaricum (Tartar Emetic)

KEYNOTES
Mucus rattling in chest, milk intolerance, nausea.

SYMPTOMS
Physical symptoms—canker sores on lips, nose fans from stuffiness. Respiratory issues feel better putting head back. Rattling in chest sound often ASSOCIATED with asthma. Better lying on right side. End-case cardio-respiratory collapse. Yawning. Vaccination reaction. Cold clammy sweat. Weak, drowsy. Any sweating.

Mental/Emotional symptoms—apathetic, weak, drowsy, irritable to noise, bad mood, wants to be alone. Child can't bear to be looked at.

MODALITIES
Worse—WARMTH, cool damp weather. Better—sitting up, coughing up mucus, motion, and cold air. Times—worse in autumn and spring, 4 P.M., cough.

ASSOCIATED
Sides—both.

Organs—diaphragm, respiratory, digestive, circulation.

Gender—masculine or feminine.

Personalities—not important.

Causation—post vaccination, anger.

Common Health Issues—asphyxia, bronchitis, emphysema, pneumonia.

APIS
Apis Mellifica (Honey Bee)

KEYNOTES
Anaphylactic shock, allergic reactions, stinging, burning, red, swelling.

SYMPTOMS
Physical symptoms—Allergy eye conditions. Swollen lower eyelids and lips, redness, skin severely swollen, puffy swelling under eyes. Insect stings, bees. Rashes from insect bites. Rashes after exercise or eating shellfish. Burns with large blisters. No thirst. Clumsy person.

Mental/Emotional symptoms—can't sit quietly, nervous, irritable, restless, hard to please. Loves to be in a family, community center. Anger. Feels neglected. Jealous women. Causeless weeping, busy.

MODALITIES
Worse—WARMTH, TOUCH, PRESSURE. Better—COLD, motion, changing position, and sitting. Time—worse at 3 to 4 P.M.

ASSOCIATED
Side—right.

Organs—mucus membranes, kidney, bladder.

Personalities—workaholics, managers, lawyers, changes jobs frequently.

Causation—allergens, bee stings, strong emotions.

Common Health Issues—allergies, bee stings, cataracts, detached retina, hives, meningitis, nephritis, rash, toxemia.

ARGENTUM NIT
Argentum Nitricum (Silver Nitrate)

KEYNOTES
PERFORMANCE ANXIETY, PANIC ATTACKS, SUGAR CRAVING.

SYMPTOMS
Physical symptoms—vertigo with trembling, nausea. Can't walk with eyes closed, unsteady. Eyes, sudden vision changes, eye tissue threatening to cover iris (pterygium). Laryngitis. Heart palpitations. Multiple Sclerosis. Warm-blooded, CRAVES SWEETS. Stomach ulcers, gastritis, gas and bloating, Crohn's disease. Green stools. Diarrhea after sweets. Right ovary problems. Can't walk correctly, uncoordinated. Old, shriveled, looks elderly, sickly.

Mental/Emotional symptoms—the performer, with performance anxiety. Hypochondriac, hysterical, nervous. Foolish gestures. Impulsive, PANIC ATTACKS, irrational, superstitious, phobic, feels forsaken. Anticipation. Speaks quickly, moving subject to subject. In a hurry, arrives early, excited, impatient. Shy, poor self-confidence.

MODALITIES
Worse—EMOTIONS, sugar, warm room, crowds, cold food, eating and drinking. Better—COLD, hard pressure, motion, wind, belching, and sitting. Time—not important.

ASSOCIATED
Sides—left.

Organs—mucus membranes, mind, nervous system, skin, bones, periosteum, larynx, right ovary.

Gender—masculine or feminine.

Personalities—students, actors, speakers, politicians, and entertainers.

Causation—anticipation, sexual excesses, SUGAR.

Common Health Issues—anticipation, depression, fears, Multiple Sclerosis, panic attacks, trembling, lack of coordination.

ARNICA
Arnica Montana (Leopard's Bane)

KEYNOTES
FIRST IN INJURIES, SHOCK, BRUISING, OVERTRAINING.

SYMPTOMS
Physical symptoms—acute or recent injuries. Red-faced, lively person. Epilepsy from injuries. Cataract from injury. Meniere's disease with vertigo. Profuse bleeding from dental injuries. Hyperventilation. Heart pain. Fatty heart degeneration. Left-sided paralysis. Bleeding, bruising, injuries of soft tissues with bruising. Fractures, stings and bites. Painful acne and small boils. Bed feels too hard. Aversion to being touched. All symptoms worse from injuries.

Mental/Emotional symptoms—irritable, angry when questioned, resists others' opinions, oversensitive to touch, sudden waking from sleep, exaggerates problems. Denies being in shock.

MODALITIES
Worse—injury, bruising, overtraining, sprains, touch, after sleep, motion, rest, damp cold, sugar, blowing nose. Better—open-air, lying low, cold bathing, changing position, sitting, wind. Time—worse sleeping.

ASSOCIATED
Sides—left.
Organs—soft tissues, temperature regulations, nerves, muscles, blood vessels.
Gender—masculine or feminine.
Personalities—athletes, manual laborers.
Causation—injuries, surgical operations, stings, bites, splinters.
Common Health Issues—aching, black eyes, blows, boils, concussion, confusion, head injury, sprains, strains, strokes, trauma.

ARSENICUM
Arsenicum Album (White Oxide of Arsenic)

KEYNOTES
OVERLY ORGANIZED, HEALTH FEARS, BURNING SENSATION, BETTER WITH HEAT.

SYMPTOMS
Physical symptoms—one may have fleshy dark skin, asthma and skin disease. Another may be lean with yellowish skin, facial wrinkles, vomiting and diarrhea. Worse-case is emaciated, older-looking, wrinkled, with diarrhea, tuberculosis, cancer, or AIDS. Canker sores (blue). ASTHMA. Unpleasant body odors, discharges. Exhaustion from diarrhea or stools, worse physical exertion. Burns, deep severe. All symptoms better HEAT. BURNING pains. Sudden weakness. THIRST. FOOD POISONING.

Mental/Emotional symptoms—Comes early, impatient, wants to know who you cured and wants to direct you, brings details. Calls back to confirm. Overly organized, miserly, selfish, restless, and health anxiety. Dependency on others for health (doctors, etc.) Preserving everything—youth, possessions, health, etc. Anxious, restless, rapid speech. Fears of disease, death of self and loved ones.

MODALITIES
Worse in cold, on exertion, midnight, drinking, infections, tobacco, eruptions. Better in warmth, motion, elevating head, sitting, and company. Time worse 10 P.M. to 12 A.M.

ASSOCIATED
Sides—right.
Organs—mucus membranes, lungs, mind, heart, spleen, skin.
Gender—masculine or feminine.
Personalities—bureaucrats, financial, precise people.
Causation—food poisoning, financial loss, poverty.
Common Health Issues—alcoholism, asthma, allergies, burning pains, food poisoning, hepatitis, kidney problems, leukemia, pneumonia, malaria.

ARSENICUM IOD
Arsenicum Iodatum (Iodide of Arsenic)

KEYNOTES
HOT, restless, allergies, irritating mucus.

SYMPTOMS
Physical symptoms—allergies with asthmatic breathing, chronic asthma. Weak heart, lungs. Tendency to diarrhea. Hard acne, HOT. Irritating discharges. Psoriasis, eczema. Wheezing (asthma), night sweats.

Mental/Emotional symptoms—RESTLESS. Overly organized. Impatient, hurried. Apathetic, wants to sit, doesn't want to interact with people. Oversensitive to noise. Worse mental effort.

MODALITIES
Worse—dry, windy, exertion, warmth, hunger, heat and cold. Better eating, rest, air flow. Time—worse 11 P.M.-2 A.M.

ASSOCIATED
Sides—left.

Organs—lungs, lymphatics, mucus membranes.

Gender—masculine or feminine.

Personalities, not important.

Causation—allergic tendencies.

Common Health Issues—allergies, asthma, emaciation, hyperactive children, lung cancer, pneumonia.

AURUM MET
Aurum Metallicum (Metallic Gold)

KEYNOTES
INTROVERTED, SUICIDAL DEPRESSION, TESTICLES, high blood pressure.

SYMPTOMS
Physical symptoms—Retinal detachment. Sensitive to pain. Hysterical, never-married women. Obese old people with heart disease. Fatty heart. High blood pressure. Angina (heart pain). Heart disease and arthritis in combination. Wringing hands. Undeveloped testicles and other right-sided testicle problems. Wandering arthritis (Pulsatilla). Sleep—moaning, bone pains at night.

Mental/Emotional symptoms—DRIVE FOR RECOGNITION. CLOSED, not revealing self. FINANCES. Needs DIGNITY, is polite. Hypochondriac, genius, introverted, serious CHILDREN, order and duty. No inner value. Can't be contradicted, wounded honor, fear of poverty, workaholic, violence causes despair. Forsaken, hopeless.

MODALITIES
Worse—emotions, mental tasks, cold, night. Better—cool, cold, warmth, motion. Times—worse sunset to sunrise.

ASSOCIATED
Sides—right.

Organs—heart, kidney, ear, testicles, bones, mind, kidneys.

Gender—masculine.

Personalities—successful business or society people.

Causation—contradiction, disappointed love, financial loss.

Common Health Issues—alcoholism, arteriosclerosis, high blood pressure, suicidal depression.

BELLADONNA
Atropa Belladonna (Deadly Nightshade)

KEYNOTES
Sudden symptoms, RED, HOT, BURNING, THROBBING, DRY, RIGHT-SIDED

SYMPTOMS
Physical symptoms—Migraine HEADACHE, right sided throbbing, right cheek red, throbbing temples. Sudden throbbing pains (headaches). RED, dilated shining PUPILS. Right eye spasms. Fevers—red, hot, throbbing, 104 to 106 degrees, dry burning-hot skin. Sunstroke. Wants lemonade. Dryness without thirst. Fatty tumors. Intelligent, vital obese people with light hair and rosy cheeks.

Mental/Emotional symptoms—jovial, entertaining, happy. Violent when ill. Delirium—wild fierce look, evil laughter, gestures, must touch everything, plays with fingers, rolls head, winks. Extroverted. Strike, bite, kick, growl. Metaphysical.

MODALITIES
Worse—heat of sun, drafts, haircuts, suppressed sweat, noise, jarring, touch, motion, cold wind, summer, stooping, warm room. Better bending backward, dark room, standing, sitting. Time—worse 3 P.M., after midnight.

ASSOCIATED
Sides—RIGHT.
Organs—brain, spine, nerves, circulation.
Gender—masculine or feminine.
Personalities—not important.
Causation—haircutting, head sweat, SUNSTROKE, drafts.
Common Health Issues—boils, delirium, delusions, earaches, hallucinations, infections, mania, mastitis, rabies, tonsillitis, vaccinations.

BELLIS
Bellis Perrennis (Daisy)

KEYNOTES
deep tissue injuries, lameness, bruising.

SYMPTOMS
Physical symptoms—injuries, blows, falls, accidents, strains, infected wounds. Used after Arnica no longer works. BOILS. Tumors, and tumors from blows. Pelvic injuries. Tailbone injury, exhausted, feels cold, worse heat. Cysts. Thirsty day and night.

Mental/Emotional symptoms—irritability, apathetic, or friendly with everyone. Neat and tidy, wants to be alone, doesn't want to talk. Identity confusion.

MODALITIES
Worse—injury, touch, sprains, cold, wet or heat. Better continued motions (Rhus tox), eating, fresh air. Times—worse sleep, 3 A.M.

ASSOCIATED
Sides—left.

Organs—circulatory, joints, nerves.

Gender—masculine or feminine.

Personalities—gardeners, construction workers.

Causation—injuries, overwork, wet exposure, childbirth.

Common Health Issues—arthritis, boils, bruises, cysts, injuries, lameness, swelling, tendonitis, tumors.

BENZOIC ACID
Benzoicum Acidum (Benzoic Acid)

KEYNOTES
strong smelling urine, GOUT, bedwetting.

SYMPTOMS
Physical symptoms—bites lower lip and sweats while eating. Asthma with arthritis, GOUT. Strong sweat odor, alternating heart and urinary issues. Wrist ganglion cyst. Strong urinary odor, dark brown and offensive. Pain Achilles tendon.

Mental/Emotional symptoms—needs and gives protection. Thinks about unpleasant things. Writing—omits words. Disgusted with deformities (compare Thuja).

MODALITIES
Worse—cold, weather change, motions, wine. Better—heat, urinating, open air. Times—not important.

ASSOCIATED
Sides—alternating sides.

Organs—URINARY, tendons, joints, heart.

Gender—masculine or feminine.

Personalities—not important.

Causation—kidney problems.

Common Health Issues—arthritis, bed wetting in children. gout, high blood pressure, Meniere's disease.

BERBERIS
Berberis Vulgaris (Barberry)

KEYNOTES
LEFT KIDNEY, KIDNEY STONES, wandering or radiating pains.

SYMPTOMS
Physical symptoms—sickly look, pale, grayish tinge, deep set eyes.
Sinusitis. Dry mucus membranes. Yellowish complexion. Gallstone
colic. Gouty pains that wander and radiate. Arthritis, prematurely old
men and women. Lives high—eats out, sleeps little, takes medications,
alcohol. Liver-related hemorrhoids and arthritis. Petechiae (red spots).
Melasma. Radiating pains, numbness, gurgling, bubbling sensation
in kidney. Sweats easily, left sinus. Cystitis, mealy sediment, cloudy.
KIDNEY STONES. HEELS, ACHILLES TENDON. Thirsty. Chilly.
Mental/Emotional symptoms—hard to think, doesn't want to talk.

MODALITIES
Worse—motion, fatigue, urinating. Better—rest, motion when in pain.
Times, not important.

ASSOCIATED
Sides—left.
Organs—left kidney, liver, mucus membranes, hips joints.
Gender—masculine or feminine.
Personalities—not important.
Causation—not known.
Common Health Issues—bladder disorders, eczema, gallstones, kidney
stones, left kidney pain, nephritis, urinary problems.

BORAX
Borax Veneta (Borate of Sodium)

KEYNOTES
tongue cankers, worse downward motion, noise sensitive.

SYMPTOMS
Physical symptoms—tangled hair. Canker sores especially on tongue. Increases milk supply in nursing mother. Pain in opposite breast nursed. DRY SKIN, poorly healing skin. Thirst increased.

Mental/Emotional symptoms—worse on unexpected noises. Shrieking in sleep. Identity confusion. Lacking borders, worse mental effort. Fears downward motion. Worse strangers. Clinging child. Cursing, delusion, is possessed. Makes space and time mistakes. Fears thunder, falling.

MODALITIES
Worse DOWNWARD or upward motion, MORNINGS, noises, cold, wet, and sleep. Better—pressure, walking open air. Times—better 11 P.M., evenings, worse mornings.

ASSOCIATED
Sides—RIGHT.

Organs—mucus membranes, mouth, urinary.

Gender—masculine or feminine.

Personalities—not important.

Causation—teething, cold wet weather.

Common Health Issues—cankers on tongue, herpes simplex, psoriasis, seasickness, thrush.

BOVISTA
Bovista Lycoperdon (Puff-Ball)

KEYNOTES
bloating, macular degeneration with bleeding.

SYMPTOMS
Physical symptoms—tension headaches. Acne from cosmetics. Macular degeneration. Thirsty. Armpits smell like garlic. Tip of tailbone itches intolerably. DRYNESS. Pressing pains. Physically awkward. Tendencies to bleeding. Everything feels enlarged. Rashes on excitement. Everything worse during menstruation or after diarrhea.

Mental/Emotional symptoms—open-hearted, moody, spatial mistakes, confused, awkward. Talkative or secretive. Confused on waking.

MODALITIES
Worse—getting warm, hot weather, eating cold food. Coffee, wine, menstruation, full moon. Better doubling up, eating, hot food. Times—worse at night

ASSOCIATED
Sides—right.

Organs—circulation, skin, nervous system.

Gender—masculine or feminine.

Personalities—not important.

Causation—carbon monoxide poisoning.

Common Health Issues—acne, carbon monoxide poisoning, colic, diarrhea, hemorrhages (excess bleeding), macular degeneration, stuttering, rashes.

BRYONIA
Bryonia Alba (Wild Hops)

KEYNOTES
SHARP PAINS WORSE WITH MOTION, DRYNESS

SYMPTOMS
Physical symptoms—dry mucus membranes, thirsty. Cankers on tip of tongue, dry tongue, moist tip. Dry hacking cough. Acute bronchial pneumonia, rib pains (Ranunculus bulb), chest trauma. Gastritis. Acute appendicitis, warm blooded. Injuries of joints, bones. Oily sweat. Sharp stitching pains. Dry, nervous, slender, irritable persons. AGGREVATION FROM MOTION, better rest.

Mental/Emotional symptoms—materialistic, talks of business. Fear of poverty, wants to be left alone. Worse thunderstorms. Hard to please.

MODALITIES
Worse—motion, exertion, heat, eating, cold, touch, during sleep. Better pressure, cold air quiet, cold water, food-belching. Times—worse morning on rising.

ASSOCIATED
Sides—RIGHT.

Organs—mucus membranes, joints, liver, chest, ribs.

Gender—masculine or feminine for pain, otherwise masculine.

Personalities—businessmen, materialistic, workaholics.

Causation—taking cold in hot weather, alcohol, injuries, cold wind.

Common Health Issues—appendicitis, arthritis, gallbladder, injuries, joint pains, lymphangitis, migraine, pleurisy, pneumonia.

CALC ARS
Calcerea Arsenicosa (Arsenite of Lime)

KEYNOTES
obesity in menopausal women, epilepsy, heart, kidney or pancreas disease.

SYMPTOMS
Physical symptoms—face goes red before epilepsy, epilepsy and heart disease combo, unusual sensation of "aura around heart." Mouth tastes like garlic, PALPITATIONS on slightest motion. Lymphatics enlarged. Family history of pancreatic cancer. Obesity of menopausal women. Prolapsed vagina during pregnancy. Anemia. Blood clots. COLD. Alcoholism. Wants SOUP.

Mental/Emotional symptoms—floating sensation, mental brilliance, fear of death (Arsenicum album), critical of others. Fears of salvation, health, future. Emotions cause heart palpitations.

MODALITIES
Worse—activity, menopause, outside, cold weather. Better—open air, rest. Times—worse nights, anxious 12-3 A.M.

ASSOCIATED
Sides—left.

Organs—pancreas, heart, nervous system, kidneys.

Gender—feminine menopausal woman. Personalities—menopausal women.

Causation—obesity in menopausal women.

Common Health Issues—anemia, epilepsy, heart disorders, heart palpitations, kidney problems, obesity in menopause, pancreas disease.

CALC CARB
Calcarea Carbonica (Carbonate of Lime)

KEYNOTES
OBESITY, OVERWORK, WEAK ANKLES, SOUR ODORS.

SYMPTOMS
Physical symptoms—weak and emaciated neck muscles, OBESITY. Knots on tip of nose. Lisping in children. SOUR SMELLS. Excessive sour sweat. Sweats into pillow at night. Chronic bronchitis. Carpal tunnel, wrist ganglion cyst. Menopause. Menstruation time worse. Polyps and bone tumors. Slow broken bone healing. NWS (never well since) OVERWORK. Everything worse from physical and mental effort. MUST SLEEP COLD (fan at night). COLD damp (clammy) feet. WEAK ANKLES.

Mental/Emotional symptoms—can't tolerate violence. Needs stability, protection, security. Lack of ambition. Lots of fears and anxiety for insanity, health, poverty, next life, animals, insects, spiders, and high places. Worries about responsibilities, duties.

MODALITIES
Worse—cold, exertion, teething, puberty, milk, clothes pressure, full moon, excess sex. Better dry weather, passing gas, dark room. Times, better morning, worse before falling asleep.

ASSOCIATED
Sides—RIGHT.

Organs—nervous system, pituitary, thyroid, parathyroid, heart, bones.

Gender—masculine or feminine.

Personalities—construction, over-workers, farmers, stone worker, sailors, thieves.

Causation—OVERWORK, poor nutrition, strains, over-lifting.

Common Health Issues—arthritis, bone problems, diabetes, epilepsy, malnutrition, osteoporosis, parasites, polyps, rickets, teething, weak ankles.

CALC FLUOR
Calcarea Fluorica (Flouride of Lime)

KEYNOTES
organs or tissues too hard or too soft, deficient tooth ENAMEL (cavities in teeth).

SYMPTOMS
Physical symptoms—pale, irregular shaped people, rickets, hyperthyroidism, tissues hard and brittle including sclerosis, scar tissue, scars. Spine problems, scoliosis. Muscle weakness.
Mental/Emotional symptoms—intellectual, depression, anxiety, indecision, fears of financial loss and poverty. Worried about health. Confused and not to the point.

MODALITIES
Worse—rest, beginning motion (Rhus tox), cold wet (damp) weather, weather change. Better—rubbing, continued motion, warmth. Time—not important.

ASSOCIATED
Sides—left.
Organs—veins, connective tissue, bones, teeth, joints, throat, thyroid.
Gender—masculine or feminine.
Personalities—critics, artists, intellectuals.
Causation—alcoholism.
Common Health Issues—bone spurs, calcification (hardening), cataracts, croup, ganglion cyst on wrist, rickets, scoliosis, deficient tooth enamel, teeth cavities, tumors, varicose veins.

CALC PHOS
Calcarea Phosphorica (Calcium phosphate)

KEYNOTES
THIN, IRRITABLE, BONE PROBLEMS, LIFE CHANGES.

SYMPTOMS
Physical symptoms—students (girls) with headaches. Long fine eye-lashes. Tendency to infections. Stiff neck. Parathyroid. Skin and bone problems. MILK intolerance. Gas. Carpal tunnel. Hip problems. Poor or excess calcification. Non-union of broken bones. Osteoporosis, sco-liosis. Sprained ankles, weak tendons and ligaments. Slow to work. Anemic children that are crabby, discontented. Fontanels close slowly in babies, teeth develop slowly. Growing pains. Craving smoked meats.

Mental/Emotional symptoms—involuntary sighing, dissatisfied, wants change, travel, low motivation, apathy. Worse with bad news. Temper tantrums worse when consoled. Moaning.

MODALITIES
Worse—weather changes, TEETHING, fluid loss, puberty, thinking of problems, menstruation. Better—warm dry weather, lying, passing gas. Times—not important.

ASSOCIATED
Sides—either.

Organs—BONES, teeth, brain, nervous system, connective tissue, chest, parathyroid.

Gender—masculine or feminine.

Personalities—artists, workaholics, job variability, truck drivers.

Causation—bone problems, disappointed in love, excessive sex.

Common Health Issues—bone problems, bone spurs, growing pains, osteoporosis, scoliosis, tobacco habits.

CALC SULPH
Calcarea Sulphurica (Gypsum, Sulphate of Lime)

KEYNOTES
Yellow, thick, lumpy pus anywhere there is an abrasion or wound, SKIN conditions.

SYMPTOMS
Physical symptoms—yellow, thick, lumpy pus from any cut or wound. Absorbs abscesses or boils. One of the top three abscess remedies, others are Silicea and Hepar sulph.

Mental/Emotional symptoms—changeable moods, evening anxiety, irritability, timid. Moody, worries about imaginary problems. Jealous.

Unusual symptoms—fear of birds and heat flushes when eating.

MODALITIES
Worse—warmth, drafts, evening, night, during sleep, menstruation, sleep. Better—bathing, washing, eating, local heat, scratching, doubling up. Times—not important.

ASSOCIATED
Sides—either.

Organs—connective tissues, SKIN, LIVER.

Gender—masculine or feminine.

Personalities—not important.

Causation—the middle child who doesn't feel appreciated, with sibling rivalry. Lack of security.

Common Health Issues—abscesses, acne (infected), pus formation, thick, yellow, lumpy pus.

CALENDULA
Calendula Officinalis (Pot Marigold)

KEYNOTES
externally use on WOUNDS, internally for WOUNDS and burns.

SYMPTOMS
Physical symptoms—externally use for burns, bites, wounds, sores. Antiseptic, prevents scarring. Internally used for exhaustion from blood loss, pain. Everything worse from fatty food. Joint and bone injuries. Takes COLD, burns, scalds, jaundice. ULCERS. PUS. Torn tendons and muscles. Broken eardrums. Bone breaks. Given before and after surgery. (Homeopathic First-Aid.)
Mental/Emotional symptoms—fears that something bad may happen. Easily frightened at small things. Sensitive to music.

MODALITIES
Worse—cloudy and damp weather. Better—lying still, warmth. Time, not important.

ASSOCIATED
Sides—either.
Organs—soft tissue, spine, liver.
Gender—masculine or feminine.
Personalities—not important.
Causation—burns or injuries.
Common Health Issues—burns, cuts, digestive ulcers, eardrums infected, injuries, surgery, puncture wounds, wounds.

CANTHARIS
Cantharis Vesicatoria (Spanish Fly)

KEYNOTES
URINARY TRACT INFECTIONS, BURNS, SUNBURN, burning stinging pains.

SYMPTOMS
Physical symptoms—red face, digestive issues with urinary problems. Sunburn. Burns (first-degree), scalds, small blisters. Muscular convulsive movements. Muscular paralysis. Inflammation of the bladder, bloody urine, scanty urine or urination upon hearing running water. Bladder leaking in pregnancy. Cystitis, URINARY TRACT INFECTIONS (UTIs), paralysis. Urinating in drops with burning, cutting pains. Constant desire to urinate. Painful stools.

Mental/Emotional symptoms—anxious, restless, hysterical especially in urinary problems. Hits, strikes, drools with rage. Or is timid confused, quarrels and fights. Sudden loss of consciousness with red face. Adultery (excess sexual desire), cursing, cruelty.

MODALITIES
Worse—urination, sound of water, coffee. Better—rubbing, warmth, rest, cold, lying on back. Times—worse at night.

ASSOCIATED
Sides—RIGHT.

Organs—urinary, genitals.

Gender—masculine or feminine.

Personalities—construction and sports.

Causation—UTI (urinary tract infection) or burns.

Common Health Issues—bladder infections, burns, hemorrhages (excess bleeding), sunburn, urinary tract infection (UTI).

CAPSICUM
Capsicum Annuum (Cayenne Pepper)

KEYNOTES
HOMESICKNESS, OBESITY, burning sensation.

SYMPTOMS
Physical symptoms—Headache with hearing loss, sensitive to noise. Eustachian tube blockage. Red nose. One red cheek. Cystitis, burning, smarting pains. Diarrhea in obese people. Cold scrotum, testicular atrophy. Obese nervous person. Older people with obesity, worse for mental work. Poor lifestyle—poor diet, no exercise. Clumsy.

Mental/Emotional symptoms—homesickness. Sleeplessness. Easily offended, critical, oppositional. Fear of slightest draft. Lazy, clumsy, sentimental. Angry. Inappropriate kissing.

MODALITIES
Worse—slight draft, cold, drinking, eating, drunkenness. Better—continued motion, heat, eating. Times—worse evenings. Both better and worse eating.

ASSOCIATED
Sides—LEFT.

Organs—ears, spleen, mucus membranes, throat.

Personalities—repetitive factory work.

Causation—homesickness.

Common Health Issues—acne, alcoholism, burning pains, homesickness, mastitis (breast infection).

CARBO VEG
Carbo Vegetabilis (Vegetable Charcoal)

KEYNOTES
GAS AND BLOATING, ICY COLD PERSON, SHOCK, EXHAUSTION.

SYMPTOMS
Physical symptoms—tip of nose, varicose veins. Thirsty during chill with cold breath. Asthma. Extreme gas, WANTS TO BE FANNED. Post-operative gas. Extremities ice cold, red. Cold body. Hemorrhages (excess bleeding) leaking persistently. Never recovered from previous illnesses. Disease has progressed to worse diseases. In last stages of disease—old face, bluing, sweaty, cold. Sluggish old people from loss of bodily fluids or injuries. Septic. Emaciation. Cold blooded. Can't wear tight clothes. SLUGGISH. Apathetic. Low energy.

Mental/Emotional symptoms—lazy, fearful, apathetic, fears of the dark, hangover. Indifference to seeing or hearing. Morning anxiety. Doesn't want company.

MODALITIES
Worse—warmth, fluid loss, exhausting disease, rich living, weather changes. Better—belching, cool air, elevating feet, being fanned. Times—worse night and in morning.

ASSOCIATED
Sides—LEFT.

Organs—circulation, GI tract, mucus membranes, heart.

Gender—masculine or feminine.

Personalities—heating and air conditioning.

Causation—carbon monoxide poisoning, blood loss, tainted or too rich foods.

Common Health Issues—asphyxia, asthma, belching, carbon monoxide poisoning, cholera, collapse, gas, heartburn, hemorrhages (excess bleeding), shock, low vitality.

CARBONEUM SULPH
Carboneum Sulphuratum (Bisulphide of Carbon)

KEYNOTES
CENTRAL VISION DISTURBANCE.

SYMPTOMS
Physical symptoms—central vision disturbances from retinal atrophy congestion. Nasal congestion. Neuralgia of teeth. Oversensitive to noise. Difficult breathing. Bad gas. Alcoholism. Periodic complaints, wants open-air. Everything worse temperature extremes. Burning or stitching pains.

Mental/Emotional symptoms—anxiety at night and morning on waking. Confusion of mind, difficult concentration, laziness. Hurried. Can't make decisions. Changeable mood.

MODALITIES
Worse—breakfast, night, motion, walking, bathing, eating. Better, open air, warm drinks. Times—worse night or on waking.

ASSOCIATED
Sides—either.

Organs—liver, eyes, nerves, mucus membranes.

Gender—masculine or feminine.

Personalities—not important.

Causation—carbon monoxide poisoning.

Common Health Issues—carbon monoxide poisoning, impotence, toothache, central vision disturbance.

CARCINOSIN
Carcinosinum (Cancer Nosode)

KEYNOTES
FAMILY CANCER HISTORY, OVERLY ORGANIZED, PASSIONATE,
LIKES TRAVEL.

SYMPTOMS
Physical symptoms—earthy face, asthma, moles, pigmentation. Cancer
history or tendency. Tics, odd types. Warm blooded. Whites of eyes are
bluish. Butter craving. Mononucleosis history. Insomnia. Cyclical vomiting alternating with diarrhea. Peptic ulcer. Gluten intolerance.

Mental/Emotional symptoms—perfectionist, sensitive, romantic, overly
organized, sympathetic to others' feelings. Sensitive to criticism. Loves
to dance. Loves animals. Wants to travel, duty-bound. Destructive children. Doesn't like authority. Fears of cancer. Rebellious as a teenager.

MODALITIES
Worse—seashore, storms, vaccinations, physical work, undressing.
Better—seashore, open-air, thunderstorms, short sleep, hot drinks.
Both worse and better by the seashore.

ASSOCIATED
Sides—either.

Organs—not important.

Gender—masculine or feminine.

Personalities—not important.

Causation—family history of cancer, sexual abuse, vaccinations.

Common Health Issues—breast cancer, diabetes, chronic fatigue, ke-
loids, gas, mononucleosis, obsessive compulsive, polyps, vaccinations.

CAUSTICUM
Causticum (Potassium Hydrate, caustic potash)

KEYNOTES
IDEALIST, PARALYSIS, URINARY LEAKAGE.

SYMPTOMS
Physical symptoms—swallowing constantly. Wrinkled forehead, Hoarseness, mornings, bronchitis. CHILLY. RIGHT FACIAL PARALYSIS. Carpal tunnel. Muscles and tendons too short. Trigger finger and finger dupuytrens contracture (Ruta graveolens). PARALYSIS with muscular atrophy. URINARY (bladder) LEAKAGE. Stool fatty and greasy. Restless legs. Tic or gestures. Burns, scalds. WARTS on hands close to nails, eyelids, tip of nose. Multiple sclerosis.

Mental/Emotional symptoms—IDEALIST, religious zealot, anarchist, protester, Robin Hood complex, yields to conscience, sympathetic to suffering of others. Fear of the dark. Overly organized. Introverted. Rigid thinking, fanaticism.

MODALITIES
Worse—COLD, DRY AIR, temperature extremes, stooping, exertion, clear weather, car riding, sweating. Better—COLD DRINKS, warmth, gentle motion, damp wet weather. Times—worse 3 to 4 A.M. or evening.

ASSOCIATED
Sides—right face, left side.

Organs—nervous system, locomotor system, muscles, and mucus membranes.

Gender—masculine or feminine.

Personalities—lawyers, politicians, idealists.

Causation—burns, scalds, worries.

Common Health Issues—Bell's Palsy, burns, facial paralysis, laryngitis, Multiple Sclerosis, muscle pains, paralysis, stuttering, strokes, tendon constriction, hoarseness or lost voice, warts.

CHAMOMILLA
Chamomilla Matricaria (German Chamomile)

KEYNOTES
TEETHING, COLIC, INTOLERABLE PAIN, WORSE ANGER, irritable children.

SYMPTOMS
Physical symptoms—nervous excitable obese people. BABY COLIC, must be carried, then refuses what's wanted. Teething, fever, and red cheeks, cough, diarrhea. Rattling mucus in chest. Belching and gas like rotten eggs. Baby restless, puts finger into mouth. Intolerance for pain, especially labor or menses. Frustration causes hepatitis, asthma. Picks bed clothes. Pregnancy—toothache, false labor.

Mental/Emotional symptoms—excessive irritability, tantrums, over-sensitivity to pain, likes being rocked, disputes authority. Crying in sleep, emotions felt in stomach.

MODALITIES
Worse—anger, teething, cold, wind, coffee, narcotics, heat, drafts, belching, dry or cloudy weather. Better—being carried, heat, sweating, fasting, warm wet weather, cold applications. Times—worse nights and mornings.

ASSOCIATED
Sides—LEFT.

Organs—nervous system, respiratory, mind, digestive, loco-motor.

Gender—feminine, children and babies.

Personalities—police and judges.

Causation—stimulant abuse-coffee or opiates, teething, bad temper.

Common Health Issues—coffee abuse, colic, teething, earaches, gas, labor disorders, menstrual disorders, severe pain, screaming.

CHIMAPHILA
Chimaphila Umbellata (Pipsissewa)

KEYNOTES
Prostate, nightly frequent urination, urinary retention, sensation as if sitting on a ball.

SYMPTOMS
Physical symptoms—prostate enlarged sensation, nightly urination, sensation as if sitting on a ball. Urination retention. Testicular atrophy or bruised sensation. Feet swelling. Kidney disease, fluttering sensation. Must stand tilted forward to urinate. Urine full of ropy mucus sediment. Kidney stones.

Mental/Emotional symptoms—feels as if sitting on a ball.

MODALITIES
Worse damp weather, cold water, sitting on cold surfaces, beginning of urination, left side. Better walking around. Time worse nighttime, better urination.

ASSOCIATED
Sides—left.

Organs—kidney, bladder, prostate, liver.

Gender—masculine or feminine.

Personalities—broken-down poor nutrition, alcoholism.

Causation—none.

Common Health Issues—alcoholism (drunk easily with beer), prostate enlargement, frequent urination, UTI (urinary tract infection).

CICUTA
Cicuta Virosa (Water Hemlock)

KEYNOTES
Convulsions, head injuries, VISION problems.

SYMPTOMS
Physical symptoms—HEAD TRAUMA, concussion. Crusty eczema on head and epilepsy. Grand mal seizures then prostration from fright. Vision problems—left half vision loss, objects move, pupils dilated, strabismus (cross eyed), photophobia. Vertigo. Stuttering speech. Cramps, spasms, rigid limbs. Muscles rigid. Craves indigestibles. Twitching and jerking. CONVULSIONS starts at stomach area in solar plexus chakra.

Mental/Emotional symptoms—objects seem too close or too far, kleptomania, wants to stay away from people. Critical, doesn't trust people, avoids people, strangers. Fear of humanity. Suspicious. Wants to be by themselves. Anxiety about future. Naive, foolish, staring, abusive.

MODALITIES
Worse—injuries, especially head, touch, noise, cold, teething, tobacco smoke, draft, jarring. Better heat, passing gas, thinking of pain. Times—not important.

ASSOCIATED
Sides—left.

Organs—brain, nerves, eyes.

Gender—masculine or feminine.

Personalities—not important.

Causation—from head injury.

Common Health Issues—concussions, convulsions, head injuries, meningitis, strabismus, tinnitus.

CIMICIFUGA
Cimicifuga Racemosa (Black Cohosh)

KEYNOTES
Neck and shoulder stiffness, depression, pessimism, hormonal—pregnancy and menopause.

SYMPTOMS
Physical symptoms—arthritis, stiff neck shoulder, trembling hands. Tongue is pointed, trembling. Arthritic. Pregnancy—fear of death, health problems, etc.; delivery, can't bear noise, shrieking in pain, hip pain and back ache; after child delivery, baby blues, painful after pains. Sighing, especially in pregnancy or menopause. Nervous urination. Cold. Delicate. Tendency to obesity. Nervous person. Hypochondriac. Hysterical.

Mental/Emotional symptoms—pessimistic (Sepia), as if dark cloud over head. Wild look. Doesn't like to answer questions or is over talkative. Sees rats or other fearful or strange objects. Suspicious. Alternates mental and physical symptoms. Nervous. Fears of insanity, especially during menstruation or menopause. Changeable.

MODALITIES
Worse—menstruation, labor, menopause, emotions, alcohol, cold damp, wind, drafts, motion, excitement. Better—warmth, pressure, continued motion, eating. Times—worse evenings mostly.

ASSOCIATED
Sides—left.
Organs—spine, muscles, uterus, ovaries, nervous system.
Gender—mostly feminine.
Personalities—grandmother, pregnant women.
Causation—emotional trauma.
Common Health Issues—arthritis, hot flashes, menopause, menstrual disorders, neck, shoulders.

CHINA/CINCHONA
China Officinalis/Cinchona Officinalis (Peruvian Bark)

KEYNOTES
INTUITIVE, never will since DEHYDRATION or fluid loss, GAS and bloating.

SYMPTOMS
Physical symptoms—obust people that are broken down from exhausting discharges and fluid losses, have become weak, sensitive and nervous. Chilly body, worse in cold. Red ear lobes. Hungry at night. Intolerant to sour Foods. Bloating. Gallstones—gallstone colic same hour worse at night. Nervous irritability and physical exhaustion. Touch irritates, hard pressure improves.

Mental/Emotional symptoms—complainers, mental and emotional irritability. INTUITIVE (Phosphorus, Sepia), sensitive, artistic. Oversensitive including touch, smell, taste. Plenty of plans and ideas. Wants only the best things. Mind—clarity at night. Feels unfortunate. Afraid of animals, violent impulses.

MODALITIES
Worse—fluid loss, light touch, noise, alternate days, cold, drafts, eating, milk, mental effort. Better—hard pressure, bending double, fasting, lying down. Times—worse night, better evening.

ASSOCIATED
Sides—left.
Organs—gallbladder, circulation, liver, blood, mucus membranes.
Gender—masculine or feminine.
Personalities—artistic, poets, journalists.
Causation—dehydration, fluids, blood loss, food poisoning.
Common Health Issues—anemia, blood loss, cirrhosis of the liver, dysentery, emaciation, food poisoning, jaundice, malaria, parasites, spleen, tinnitus (ringing in ears).

CLEMATIS
Clematis Erecta (Virgin's Bower)

KEYNOTES
TOBACCO ADDICTION, problems from sexualy-transmitted diseases when treated with antibiotics, neuralgic pains, hardened glands.

SYMPTOMS
Physical symptoms—Glands swollen. Toothache from tobacco, worse at night. TOBACCO ADDICTION. Right testicular pain. Problems from gonorrhea and antibiotic treatment. Avoids sex. Hard to urinate. Electrical shock pains lying down.

Mental/Emotional symptoms—apathy, no willpower, no joy. Thoughts of dying. Homebody, weeping, foggy thinking, sleepiness, confused—better in open-air.

MODALITIES
Worse—gonorrhea, night, heat of bed, tobacco smoke, moving head. Better sweating, scratching, open-air. Times—worse mornings, waking, 3 to 5 P.M.

ASSOCIATED
Sides—LEFT.

Organs—mucus membranes, genitals, male, female.

Gender—masculine or feminine.

Personalities—sexually transmitted diseases treated with antibiotics.

Causation—homesickness.

Common Health Issues—eye problems, gonorrhea, infections, right testicle, toothaches.

COCCULUS
Cocculus Indicus (Indian Cockle)

KEYNOTES
#1 MOTION SICKNESS, CARETAKER, neurological diseases.

SYMPTOMS
Physical symptoms—head, hollow sensation. weak neck. Vertigo, seasickness, car sickness, MOTION SICKNESS. Cold breasts. Numb hands. Weak abdominal muscles. Severe muscle cramps. COLDNESS. Sleep, shrieking, open eyes. Degenerative neurological disorders, MS (Multiple Sclerosis, ALS, Alzheimer's—with leg paralysis. Extreme weakness. CARETAKERS. Weak abdominal muscles. Everything worse traveling. Timid nervous persons. Picks at bed clothes. Strange body positions. Bookworms (Nat Mur).

Mental/Emotional symptoms—serious, INTROVERTED, sensitive, timid. Nervous teen girls, unmarried women, or childless. Oversensitive, slowness in comprehension, worries, confused after eating or drinking. Time passes too quickly. ROMANTIC. Doesn't like to be contradicted, wants to sing.

MODALITIES
Worse—traveling, boat or car, loss of sleep, cold, anxiety, food smells, drinking coffee, pregnancy, laughing, crying. Better—quiet warm room. Time—worse sleep loss.

ASSOCIATED
Sides—right, one-sided.

Organs—SENSES, SPINE.

Gender—feminine, women and girls.

Personalities—pilots, nurses, shift workers.

Causation—nursing mothers, sleep loss, motion sickness.

Common Health Issues—chronic fatigue, motion sickness, muscle weakness, nursing mothers, sleep deprivation, vertigo, vomiting.

COFFEA
Coffea Cruda (Unroasted Coffee)

KEYNOTES
OVERACTIVE MIND, SLEEPLESSNESS due to busy mind-mind racing, OVERSENSITIVE SENSES.

SYMPTOMS
Physical symptoms—coffee or caffeine headaches. Sleeplessness from mental activity. Toothache better from ice. TEETHING with hypersensitive female genitals, acute sense of smell, asthmatic breathing. Sensitivity to noise hearing, or music. MENOPAUSE.

Mental/Emotional symptoms—excessive emotions, overactive mind, delusions of floating. Quick to act, humorous, over sensitivity of pain. Senses overactive. Things seem very pleasurable, is over-alert. Tossing about in anguish, fear of death from pain.

MODALITIES
Worse—noise, touch, odors, air, mental effort, overeating, emotions, cold, narcotics. Better—lying, rest, ice water in mouth. Time—worse at night.

ASSOCIATED
Sides—right.

Organs—nerves, circulation, mind, sexual organs.

Gender—feminine.

Personalities—not important.

Causation—sudden emotions, especially pleasurable.

Common Health Issues—colic, excitement, insomnia, labor pains, sleeplessness, toothaches, unconsciousness.

COLCHICUM
Colchicum Autumnale (Meadow Saffron)

KEYNOTES
GOUT, SENSITIVE TO SMELL.

SYMPTOMS
Physical symptoms—oversensitive to odors, cooking, etc., bright lights, noise, pain, touch. Gag from mention or smell of food. LIVER disorders. Gout of big toe, joints. Edema, swelling due to kidney weakness. Ailments from radiation therapy. Weakness, doesn't want to be disturbed. Better not moving.

Mental/Emotional symptoms—sensitive to rude people, loss of spatial perception, confused, oversensitive in general.

MODALITIES
Worse—motion, weather, cold damp, Autumn, sundown to sunrise, loss of sleep, heat, STRONG ODORS. Better—warmth, rest, lying quiet, sitting still. Time—worse at night, 11 P.M. to 3 A.M. especially asthma.

ASSOCIATED
Sides—left or left to right.

Organs—digestive, heart, kidneys, muscles, joints.

Gender—masculine or feminine.

Personalities—not important.

Causation—emotional trauma, caretaking, suppressed sweat.

Common Health Issues—arthritis, diarrhea, gas, gout, morning sickness, MS (Multiple Sclerosis, 40 percent of cases), nausea, vomiting.

COLOCYNTHIS
Citrullus Colocynthis (Bitter Cucumber)

KEYNOTES
COLON pain or other PAIN FROM ANGER or FRUSTRATION. Better heat and pressure or doubling over.

SYMPTOMS
Physical symptoms—tri-facial neuralgia (facial nerve pain). Bitter taste in mouth. Sweat smells like urine. Obesity. Below bellybutton pain as if smashed between rocks. Sedentary women with heavy menstruation. Mucusy stool with musty odor. Muscle spasms from anger. Sciatica right side. Twisting and tearing pain. Pains worse anger or frustration. Everything better doubling over, warmth, lying on belly.

Mental/Emotional symptoms—irritable, frustrated, contorted face, screams, throws things. Anger causes pain, cramping and restlessness. Depressed and joyless. Affected by others' tragedies.

MODALITIES
Worse—frustration, anger, draft, cold, cheese, lying or motion. Better doubling over, hard pressure, coffee, touch, stool, passing gas. Time—worse night and 4 to 5 P.M.

ASSOCIATED
Sides—RIGHT.

Organs—GI tract, nerves, genitals.

Gender—masculine or feminine.

Personalities—not important.

Causation—frustration, business failure, excess sex.

Common Health Issues—colic, intestinal cramps, ovarian cysts—right; menstrual pains, sciatica—right.

CONIUM
Conium Maculatum (Poison Hemlock)

KEYNOTES
PROSTATE or BREAST problems, CANCER, MATERIALISTIC.

SYMPTOMS
Physical symptoms—menopause. Double vision or other vision problems, photophobia. Lots of earwax. Swollen lymph glands or cancerous. Stony hard lymphatic glands. Painful breasts enlarged before menstruation. Breast cancer. Mastitis. Lung cancer nodule. Picks or plays with fingers. Ascending paralysis (starts in lower body and moves up). Used to lower male PSA. Prostate cancer. Elderly man, no sex for a long time or is celibate. Fashionista woman with rich clothes, not taken care of (unkempt). Slow passive people, inflexible, irritable.

Mental/Emotional symptoms—apathetic, introverted, conservative, celibate, overly organized, attached to material things, sex or are sober, severe grief, suppressed sexual desire.

MODALITIES
Worse—alcohol, appearance of moving objects, masturbation, cold, milk, motion. Better pressure, fasting, continued motion (Rhus tox), sitting down. Time—worse at night.

ASSOCIATED
Sides—RIGHT.

Organs—glands, nerves, muscles, breast, prostate.

Gender—masculine or feminine.

Personalities—priests, materialists.

Causation —wounds, sexual excess, celibacy.

Common Health Issues—breast cancer, cervical problems, injuries, MS, muscle weakness, prostate cancer, trembling.

CROCUS
Crocus Sativa* (Saffron)

KEYNOTES
SEVERE BLEEDING, dark stringy black blood.

SYMPTOMS
Physical symptoms—nosebleeds in hot weather, stringy blood, black. Nosebleeds instead of menstruation. Bleeding long black stringy blood. Old open scars bleed. Severe constipation. Wants open air. Sensation as if something living in the abdomen. Sleep—laugh, sings, shrieks, walking in. Hysteric, weak, nervous women. Mental and physical symptoms alternate.

Mental/Emotional symptoms—jesting, talkative. Increased sexual desire. Wants to kiss everyone then gets angry. Quick changes of mood. Immoderate laughter, manic or silly. Childish—foolish, spastic laughing, loves cheerful music.

MODALITIES
Worse—motion, pregnancy, menstruation, puberty, reading, fasting, warm room, lying down. Better open air, after breakfast. Time—worse mornings.

ASSOCIATED
Sides—left.

Organs—capillary system, eyes, nerves, female organs, mind.

Gender—feminine, women and children.

Personalities—not important.

Causation—effects of blows or injury.

Common Health Issues—constipation, hemorrhages (excess bleeding), nosebleeds.

*Not in found in conditions chapter.

CROTALUS HORR
Crotalus Horridus (Rattle Snake)

KEYNOTES
Hemorrhages (excess bleeding) when Phosphorus doesn't work. It looks like a right-sided Lachesis.

SYMPTOMS
Physical symptoms—sallow face, jaundice. Eye, retinal hemorrhages (excess bleeding). Bleeding gums. Trembling tongue. Nosebleed. Tight chest. Bleeding. Heart problems in menopause. Pain extending to left hand. Infections. Menstrual hemorrhages. Menopausal hot flashes. Cold body with hot flashes. All symptoms worse hunger, alcohol, and tight clothes (Lachesis).

Mental/Emotional symptoms—social, extrovert, but aversion to family members. Mumbling, talkative (Lachesis). Sensitive. Dictatorial, irritable. Delusions of being surrounded by enemies. Suspicious, talks of death.

MODALITIES
Worse—alcohol, right side, spring, physical exertion, cold dry air. Better—rest, motion, waking. Time—worse on waking.

ASSOCIATED
Sides—RIGHT.

Organs—BLOOD, CIRCULATION, nerves, liver.

Gender—masculine or feminine.

Personalities—not important.

Causation—vaccines, fright, alcohol.

Common Health Issues—Bubonic plague, cirrhosis of the liver, edema (swelling), hemorrhages (excess bleeding), jaundice, paralysis, plague, blood poisoning, stroke, yellow fever.

CUPRUM MET
Cuprum Metallicum (Copper)

KEYNOTES
CRAMPS, SPASMS, SYMPTOMS WORSE NIGHT.

SYMPTOMS
Physical symptoms—distorted bluish face and lips. Bluish marbled skin. Stuttering, convulsions in teething children. Hyperthyroid (overactive thyroid). Cough gurgling sound. Spasms, convulsions, falls, shrieks. Thumbs clenched. Jerks up in bed, sleeps on stomach. mentally and physically exhausted from mental work or sleep deprivation.

Mental/Emotional symptoms—compulsive neurosis, reserved while speaking. Serious, critical, guilty, responsible—full of duty. Self-disciplined or lack thereof, can be ambitious. Spitting, headstrong, seductive, plays the fool.

MODALITIES
Worse—suppressed eruptions, motion, hot weather, cold, pregnancy, raising arms. Better—pressure on heart, sweating, cold drinks. Time—worse at night.

ASSOCIATED
Sides—left.

Organs—nervous system, muscles, blood.

Gender—masculine or feminine.

Personalities—singers with occasional loss of voice.

Causation—suppressed eruptions.

Common Health Issues—cholera, convulsions, cramps, epilepsy, meningitis, spasms, whooping cough.

DIGITALIS
Digitalis Purpurea* (Foxglove)

KEYNOTES
SLOW PULSE, palpitations on least movement, HEART and LIVER DISEASE.

SYMPTOMS
Physical symptoms—retinal detachment. Blue veins appear on eyes, ears, lips, tongue. Chest constriction. Heart failure, heart enlarged, heart mitral valve problems. SLOW PULSE. Heart palpitations least movement. Fears to move as if heart would cease to beat. Caused by scarlet or rheumatic fever. Wants bitter foods. Liver enlarged. Liver problems with diarrhea and heart disease. Skin itching, jaundice or yellow. Needs to urinate. Prostatic enlargement in old men. Dropsy—swelling. Anxious, nervous, elderly women with brown complexion.

Mental/Emotional symptoms—cardiac problems from unhappy love affair. Grief, disappointment, fear of failure, wants to run away. Fear of death from heart disease. Deep sighing. Music makes sad. Dreams of falling (mostly women). Obstinate.

MODALITIES
Worse—physical exertion, rising up, heat, lying on left side, motion, smells of food, sexual excess, talking, excitement, music. Better—empty stomach, rest, cool air, fasting, pressure, weeping, urination. Time—worse at night, worse on waking.

ASSOCIATED
Sides—right.
Organs—HEART, liver, stomach, circulation, genital, urinary.
Gender—masculine or feminine.
Personalities—not important.
Causation—High, rich living, alcoholism, sexual abuse.
Common Health Issues—cyanosis (blueness), difficult breathing, heart mitral valve, heart pain, heart disorders, hot flashes, prostate enlargement, urethritis.
*Not found in Conditions chapter.

DROSERA
Drosera Rotundifolia (Sundew)

KEYNOTES
WHOOPING COUGH or SPASMODIC COUGH, laryngitis.

SYMPTOMS
Physical symptoms—yellow mucus. Hoarseness, laryngitis, deep voice. Asthma when talking. Chronic bronchitis with burning in chest. Harsh spasmodic cough. Fever with whooping cough. Sweats easily. Pains in long bones. Coughing bloody mucus. Stiff, inflexibility of ankles. Children—failure to thrive, malnourished, starving. Growing pains in children. Cold body.

Mental/Emotional symptoms—mistrustful, feels deceived. Sadness about the future. Anxiety when alone. Hard to concentrate. Over talkative. Anxious, restless. Obstinate. Feels forsaken. Homesick. Discouraged.

MODALITIES
Worse—lying down, warmth, singing, crying, rest, applying pressure. Better—sitting up, walking, motion, being quiet. Times—worse at midnight.

ASSOCIATED
Sides—right.

Organs—respiratory, bones, larynx.

Gender—masculine or feminine.

Personalities—not important. Causation—family history of tuberculosis.

Common Health Issues—asthma, bronchitis, coughs, laryngitis, tuberculosis, whooping cough, writer's cramp.

DULCAMARA
Solanum Dulcamara (Woody Nightshade)

KEYNOTES
COLD DAMP CONDITIONS, FUNGAL SKIN PROBLEMS, WARTS.

SYMPTOMS
Physical symptoms—dandruff. Pale face with red cheeks. Seizures start in face, speechless—mouth drawn to one side. Herpes on lips. Tonsillitis from change of weather. Mucus yellow. Asthma from damp cool conditions—autumn. OBESITY. Bellybutton pain. WARTS, large, flat, smooth, of the palms and fingers. Fungal skin problems (Thuja). Skin problem with thick crust. Ringworm (Tellurium). Diarrhea from catching cold. Stamps the feet. Coldness in painful parts. Everything worse COLD WET WEATHER.

Mental/Emotional symptoms—quarrelsome, scolding, domineering, grumbling. Impatient in the morning.

MODALITIES
Worse—chilled, cold wet, sweating, eruptions, menstruation, autumn, night, before storms. Better—motion, walking, warm, dry weather. Time—not significant.

ASSOCIATED
Sides—left.

Organs—mucus membranes, skin, lower back.

Gender—masculine or feminine.

Personalities—Cold-storage workers.

Causation—COLD DAMP CONDITIONS.

Common Health Issues—arthritis, colds, glandular swelling, mononucleosis, nasal congestion, sore throat, neck stiff, rashes, warts, herpes on lips.

EQUISETUM
Equisetum Hyemale (Horsetail)

KEYNOTES
BEDWETTING, URINARY TRACT INFECTIONS, BLADDER.

SYMPTOMS
Physical symptoms—frowny face. Increased appetite. Bedwetting. Urinary tract infections. Kidneys feel heavy, dull pain right side. Bladder feels full, distended, urging, painful after urination. Urine cloudy with mucus, or large quantities of light-colored gritty urine. Sharp burning pains. Frequent night urination. Ailments from abuse of diuretics. Everything is better in the afternoon.

Mental/Emotional symptoms—irritable, exhausted, dreams of crowds of people. Nightmares with bedwetting.

MODALITIES
Worse—right side, movement, touch, sitting, finishing urinating. Better—afternoon, lying down, continued motion. Time—bedwetting after just getting to asleep.

ASSOCIATED
Sides—right.

Organs—urinary tract.

Gender—masculine or feminine.

Personalities—not important.

Causation—diuretic abuse or chronic use of diuretics.

Common Health Issues—bedwetting, incontinence, frequent urination, kidney problems, diuretic abuse.

EUPHRASIA
Euphrasia Officinalis (Eyebright)

KEYNOTES
BURNING TEARS, EXCESS EYE MUCUS, EYE REMEDY.

SYMPTOMS
Physical symptoms—eye problems. IRRITATING TEARS, burning and smarting. Excess tears. Tears in cold air, headaches with wind irritation. Eye injuries. Red eyes. Styes. Conjunctivitis (inflammation of inner eyelids). Hair in eyes sensation. Lots of blinking. Bland nasal mucus discharges. Allergies (hay fever)—irritating sinus discharges. Head cold. All symptoms worse upon waking.
Mental/Emotional symptoms—irritation from eye problems.

MODALITIES
Worse—evening, sunlight, wind, touch, morning. Better—wiping eyes, open air, low light. Time—worse in the evening, and morning.

ASSOCIATED
Sides—more left, some right.
Organs—Eyes, nose, mucus membranes.
Gender—masculine or feminine.
Personalities—computer techs or detail work.
Causation—dusty wind, allergies, excess reading or computer work.
Common Health Issues—allergies, conjunctivitis, measles, excess tears, weak eyes from computer work.

FERRUM MET
Ferrum Metalicum (element Iron)

KEYNOTES
ANEMIA, PALE, HEMORRHAGES (EXCESS BLEEDING), better walking slowly.

SYMPTOMS
Physical symptoms—pale (anemic) or dirty skin (excess iron). Flushed face, worse stooping. Nosebleeds in children. Goiter. Arthritis—left shoulder. Large appetite. Can't tolerate eggs. Obese or emaciated people. Heavy menstruation. Ulcerative colitis. Nightly diarrhea. Coughing from tobacco smoke. Feels better when distracted. Wants to be fanned. Feels better walking around slowly. Excess iron supplement use.

Mental/Emotional symptoms—combative, domineering, can't hear contradiction, unyielding, must have the last word. Wants solitude. Worries about family. Moody. Oversensitive to noise. Ailments from anger.

MODALITIES
Worse—night, emotions, fluid loss, sweating, being still, overheating, menstruation. Better—slow-moving, summer, pressure, being by self. Time—worse at night.

ASSOCIATED
Sides—left.

Organs—circulation, BLOOD, GI tract, digestion.

Gender—feminine.

Personalities—not important.

Causation—blood loss.

Common Health Issues—anemia, arthritis, blood problems, constipation, hemorrhage, miscarriage, morning sickness.

FERRUM PHOS
Ferrum Phosphoricum (Iron phosphate)

KEYNOTES
bleeding, fever, anemia, inflammation.

SYMPTOMS
Physical symptoms—eye, conjunctivitis. Transparent skin. Paleness alternating with redness. painful acute earaches. Nosebleeds. Facial neuralgia (nerve pain) better by cold application. White mucus discharges. Colds and flu (alternate with Kali mur). Fevers of 99-101 degrees. Mucus, rattling in chest (Antimonium tart). Joint pains. Anemia, or excess blood iron, first remedy. Hemochromatosis (excessive iron). Nervous, sensitive, pale or anemic persons. Sleep with eyes half-open. After-surgery soreness.

Mental/Emotional symptoms—mental exhaustion, feels hurried, wants to protect others, excited about life. Anxiety after eating or being confused. Spontaneous behavior. Indifferent about life.

MODALITIES
Worse—cold or open-air, right side, motion, noise, cold drinks, sour food. Better—cold application, bleeding, lying down, gentle motion. Time—worse from 4 to 6 A.M., and night.

ASSOCIATED
Sides—right.
Organs—circulation, lungs, eustachian tubes, blood.
Gender—masculine or feminine.
Personalities—singers.
Causation—blood loss, or injury.
Common Health Issues—first onset cold or flu, ear eustachian-tube blockage, fevers, hemorrhages (excess bleeding), tonsillitis.

FLUORIC ACID
Fluoricum Acidum (Hydrofluoric Acid)

KEYNOTES
TEETH, BONES, MATERIALISTIC.

SYMPTOMS
Physical symptoms—hair dry, falls out. Transparent skin. Deep cracks in tongue. Teeth discolored, crumbling, deficient enamel, cavities. Goiter. Desires spicy foods. Emaciation. Crumbling nails. Scars. Warts close to nails. Bone weakness. Peyronies (curved penis). Sweaty genitals. Swollen scrotum. Weak constitutions. Water retention. Masculine women. Young people look old. Hot-blooded (Sulphur).

Mental/Emotional symptoms—shocks others, egotists, materialistic, no sense of responsibility. Superficial relationships, sexually promiscuous at a young age. Odd gesturing, bad temper. Psychosis, overconfident, opinionated, sexually precocious, looking to take advantage of others.

MODALITIES
Worse—heat, alcohol, night. Better—cold washing, open cool air, eating, urination, bending backwards, rapid movement. Time—worse at night.

ASSOCIATED
Sides—right.

Organs—connective tissue, varicose veins.

Gender—masculine or feminine.

Personalities—successful business people.

Causation—fluoride deficiency.

Common Health Issues—bone problems, digestive ulcers, edema-swelling, fluoride poisoning, goiter, teeth problems, varicose veins.

GELSEMIUM
Gelsemium Sempervirens (Yellow Jasmine)

KEYNOTES
FRIGHT, PANIC ATTACKS, TREMORS, CHRONIC FATIGUE, SHOCK.

SYMPTOMS
Physical symptoms—dull, stupid expression on face. Flushed face. Eyes, detached retina, astigmatism, strabismus (cross-eyed). Double vision. Vertigo. Pulse slow, in the elderly. Weakness with paralysis. Slow developing INFLUENZA, FLU. Tremors. Trembling. Drowsy, apathetic.

Mental/Emotional symptoms—nervous women. Anticipation, PANIC ATTACKS, shuts down. Poor willpower, fear of losing control. Fears that heart will stop beating. Stage fright with diarrhea and urging to urinate. Doesn't want to be disturbed. Apathy towards their illness.

MODALITIES
Worse—emotions, excitement, shock, cold damp (spring), thinking of ailments, tobacco. Better—urination, sweating, shaking, alcohol, mental work, bending forward. Time—not important.

ASSOCIATED
Sides—right.

Organs—nervous system, eyes, mucus membranes.

Gender—especially feminine.

Personalities—artists, students.

Causation—fright, shock, drug or alcohol abuse, masturbation.

Common Health Issues—anxiety, bad news, chronic fatigue, double vision, drug overdose, fright, influenza, muscle weakness, paralysis, tremors, vertigo, weakness.

GLONOINUM
Glonoinum (Nitro-Glycerine)

KEYNOTES
Migraines that throb to the beat of the heart, SUNSTROKE.

SYMPTOMS
Physical symptoms—blood rushes to head and causes violent throbbing to the beat of the heart on the right side. Pulsating pain between temples. Heat in head. Frontal headache with sweating, worse with motion. Red face comes and goes. Sunstroke. All symptoms worse in warm air, sun exposure, and MENOPAUSE.

Mental/Emotional symptoms—confusion due to head congestion. Fear of choking. Staring or wild expression. Time passes too slowly. Aversion to family, worse quarreling. Confusion. Dwells on offenses of the past.

MODALITIES
Worse—heat, sun, weather, motion, pressure on head, haircut, rising up from sitting. Better—open-air, raising head, cool, pressure, application. Time—worse 6 A.M. to noon.

ASSOCIATED
Sides—right.

Organs—head, circulation, brain, heart.

Gender—masculine or feminine.

Personalities—not important.

Causation—sunstroke, emotions, angina (heart pain).

Common Health Issues—angina (heart pain), Basedow's disease, migraines, heart palpitations, strokes, sunstroke.

GRAPHITES
Graphites Naturalis (Black Lead)

KEYNOTES
OBESITY, KELOID SCARS, AND OTHER SKIN ISSUES, NO SEX DRIVE.

SYMPTOMS
Physical symptoms—eyes, photophobia. Pasty look. Large cheeks. Swollen glands. Earaches—left side. Deep skin cracks behind the ears, oozing. Swollen lymphatics. Sweating while talking, especially behind the ears. Anemia. Breast problems including abscess or cancer. Obesity. Chilly body. Big hands. Skin rough, hard, and dry with deep cracks oozing a honey-like discharge (behind ears too). Skin problems with pus. Keloid (raised) scars. Reiter's syndrome (arthritis, conjunctivitis, and urethritis together). Menopause. Masculine women with scanty menstrual flow and profuse vaginal discharge. Constipated. Stools, lumpy with mucus. Anal deep skin cracks. Toes swollen.

Mental/Emotional symptoms—dull, lethargic, slow—can't make up mind. Timid. Can't logically think, worried about future problems. Overly organized. Weepy, music makes better. Anxiety on waking. NO SEX DRIVE. Restless while working. Obstinate and Moody. Periodic depression.

MODALITIES
Worse—cold, draft, menstruation, eating fats, physical exertion, hot drinks, music, wet feet. Better—walking, eating, touch, no noise, belching, car driving. Time—worse before midnight.

ASSOCIATED
Sides—LEFT.
Organs—skin folds, skin, circulation, lymphatics, eyes.
Gender—masculine or feminine.
Personalities—construction, truck driver, farmer.
Causation—from grief, over lifting, surgery.
Common Health Issues—eczema, fissures (deep skin cracks), GI (digestive) problems, nail problems, obesity, heart palpitations, psoriasis, scars, tissue or skin hardening, skin problems, vaginal discharges (leuchorrhea).

HAMAMELIS
Hamamelis Virginiana (Witch Hazel)

KEYNOTES
HEMORRHAGES (EXCESS BLEEDING), passive bleeding (flows slowly, seeping), soreness.

SYMPTOMS
Physical symptoms—headache left temple, left eye. Eye bleeds with iritis. Black eye from being bruised. Bleeding gums. Great thirst. Nosebleeds. Passive bleeding (flows out slowly, seeping). Profuse bleeding—passive injuries. Exhaustion from slight bleeding. Skin, first degree burns. Women, heavy menstruation. Menstruation with abdominal soreness. Pregnancy with painful varicose veins on legs and vulva. Birthing with passive bleeding, hemorrhoids, sore nipples. Bleeding varicose veins. Hard knotty veins. Aching pain. Sore pain. Bruised soreness. All symptoms worse with touch.

Mental/Emotional symptoms—wants to be respected. Tranquility with hemorrhage. Must think quietly.

MODALITIES
Worse from injuries, bruises, jarring, motion, exertion, moist air. Time—worse night.

ASSOCIATED
Sides—not important.

Organs—veins and venous circulation, ovaries, liver.

Gender—masculine or feminine.

Personalities—not important.

Causation—not important.

Common Health Issues—aching, bruising, burns, hemorrhages (excess bleeding), hemorrhoids, phlebitis (vein inflammation), varicose ulcers, varicose veins.

HELLEBORUS
Helleborus Niger (Snow-rose)

KEYNOTES
HEAD INJURIES with indifference to loved ones.

SYMPTOMS
Physical symptoms—brain injury. Sleep after brain injury or surgery. Head injury leads to mental dullness, sleepiness, slowness. Rattling in throat. Gradual mental decline, rolls head and moans, buries head in pillow (ESPECIALLY CHILDREN). Automatic motion of one arm and leg. COLD body. Wandering pains.

Mental/Emotional symptoms—stupor, slowness of thinking, dull sensation, has to concentrate. Apathy. Homesickness. Involuntary sighing. Hopelessness, despair.

MODALITIES
Worse—puberty, cold air, teething, uncovering. Better—distraction, open-air. Time—worse from 4 to 8 P.M., evening to morning as well.

ASSOCIATED
Sides—left.

Organs—brain, nervous system, mucus membranes, muscles.

Gender—masculine or feminine.

Personalities—not important.

Causation—concussion, head injury, or love loss.

Common Health Issues—brain injuries, coma, concussions, meningitis, night blindness.

HEPAR SULPH
Hepar Sulphuris Calcareum (Calcium Sulphide)

KEYNOTES
Thick, yellow-green pus, smells of old cheese, splinter-like pains, sensitive to drafts.

SYMPTOMS
Physical symptoms—sour smell, thick pus from infections or wounds with inflamed red borders. Infected skin injuries. All discharges smell like old cheese. Low pain threshold, splinter-like pains. Excessive sour bad-smelling sweat. Feels cold.

Mental/Emotional symptoms—emotional. Fast speech. Irritable, sour tempered, easily offended or upset. Impulsive. Threatening violence. Pyromaniac, feels the world is on fire. Feels vulnerable.

MODALITIES
Worse—cold dry air, draft, night. Better—moist damp heat, damp weather or dry winds. Time—not important.

ASSOCIATED
Sides—right.

Organs—skin, nerves, respiratory, lymphatic system.

Gender—masculine or feminine.

Personalities—not important.

Causation—cold dry winds, injuries, suppressed skin conditions using steroid creams.

Common Health Issues—pus caused from injury or infection process, abscesses, boils, skin problems.

HYOSCYAMUS
Hyoscyamus Niger* (Henbane)

KEYNOTES
EROTIC BEHAVIOR, OBESITY, SPASMS.

SYMPTOMS
Physical symptoms—pale or bluish face. Bites tongue when talking. Stuttering, trembling tongue. Bulimia. Odd gestures, must touch everything, Worse when touched. Obesity. Muscles spasm, twitch, jerk. Sleeps naked; walking, talking, moaning, weeping, smiling, laughing, grinding teeth during sleep. Seizure-like symptoms with clenched fist, retracted thumbs, twitching, crying, anxiety. Dresses indecently—low neckline, short skirts (Platina).

Mental/Emotional symptoms—hysterical, nervous, excitable. Loquacity (talkative). Stares. Picks at fingers. Shameless exhibitionist—cursing, obscene, sexual antics, especially in teens. Psychosis, jealous, suspicious, rocking to and fro. Violence, self-mutilation, threatens to kill others.

MODALITIES
Worse—emotions, touch, menstruation, eating and drinking, sleep, rest. Better—stooping, sitting up. Time—worse sleep.

ASSOCIATED
Sides—left.

Organs—brain, nervous system, mind, blood.

Gender—masculine or feminine.

Personalities—prostitutes, transvestites, actors, singers, priests.

Causation—grief, love lost, jealousy, fright.

Common Health Issues—alcoholism, delirium, hysteria, insanity, mania, mental disorders, nymphomania (hypersexuality), senility.

*Not found in Conditions chapter.

HYPERICUM PERF
Hypericum Perforatum (St. John's Wort)

KEYNOTES
NERVE INJURIES, SHOOTING PAINS, TAILBONE INJURIES.

SYMPTOMS
Physical symptoms—headache from spinal tap. Forceps injury at birth. Facial neuralgia and toothache. Toothache after dental work or injury. Asthma after spinal injuries. Obesity. Nerve injuries, fingers, toes, fingernails. Nerve spasms. Jerking and twitching muscles. Pinched nerves. Shooting pains along nerves. Pain intolerable. Puncture wounds, bites, tetanus. Tailbone injuries. Pain in tailbone during and after childbirth.

Mental/Emotional symptoms—hurried. Depressive mood. Makes mistakes in speaking, writing. Complaints from fright or shock.

MODALITIES
Worse—injury, jarring, shock, change of weather, cold damp, motion, cold air. Better—quietude, bending backward, lying on stomach. Time—not important.

ASSOCIATED
Sides—either.

Organs—brain, nervous system, lower spine, tailbone.

Gender—masculine or feminine.

Personalities—not important.

Causation—nerve injuries, dental work.

Common Health Issues—bites, blood poisoning, injuries, neuralgia, spinal cord injuries, spine injuries, tailbone injuries, tetanus, wounds.

Ignatia

IGNATIA
Ignatia Amara (St. Ignatius Bean)

KEYNOTES
SIGHING, HYSTERICAL CRYING, GRIEVING, LUMP IN THROAT.

SYMPTOMS
Physical symptoms—tongue trembles. Globus hystericus (lump in the throat). Vitiligo (loss of skin pigment). Hirsutism (dark, thick, coarse hair on face in women, sometimes chest) (Lycopodium, Sepia, Thuja). Hands tremble in other's presence. Thin sensitive, excitable women. Masculine look, exotic clothing, reserved, aloof, guarded, exaggerated sickness, silly or forced laughter or cheerfulness. All symptoms worse tobacco, smoke.
Mental/Emotional symptoms—sighing. Delicate, romantic, emotional, from a recent shock or grief. Emotional outbursts with crying. Eats from stress. Worse for consolation. High expectations, resentment, bitter feelings. Exaggeration of sickness. History of incest.

MODALITIES
Worse—emotions, odors, touch or slight touch, tobacco, consolation, winter. Better—urination, hard pressure, swallowing, being alone. Time—worse on waking.

ASSOCIATED
Sides—RIGHT.
Organs—nervous system, mind, emotions.
Gender—mostly feminine.
Personalities—pianist, artists.
Causation—DISAPPOINTED LOVE or other emotional losses.
Common Health Issues—amenorrhea (lack of menstruation), colic, convulsions, depression, disappointment, grief, hysteria, heart palpitations, sighing, tremors, twitching, parasites, worry.

IPECAC
Cephaelis Ipecacuanha (Ipecac-root)

KEYNOTES
NAUSEA OR VOMITING with a clean tongue, excessive saliva, dry heaves, stomach sinking sensation, MORNING SICKNESS.

SYMPTOMS
Physical symptoms—dark circles under eyes. Nausea on looking at moving objects with excessive saliva. Tongue clean with nausea and vomiting, stomach sinking sensation. Dry heaving. Vomiting worse stooping. MORNING SICKNESS. Coughing, dry and gagging, may end up vomiting. Respiratory issues with nausea and vomiting, bleeding from lungs. Bright red blood in any hemorrhage (excess bleeding) with nausea. Diarrhea in autumn. Fat, feeble children. Flabby adults. Opiate addiction.

Mental/Emotional symptoms—hard to please, disagreeable, frustrated, feels unfortunate, life is hard, noise intolerance. Ailments from suppressed anger, jealous.

MODALITIES
Worse—warm and damp, overeating, motion, autumn, opiates. Better—open air. Time—not important.

ASSOCIATED
Sides—right.

Organs—GI tract, stomach, nerves, vagus nerve, mucus membranes, respiratory.

Gender—masculine or feminine.

Personalities—not important.

Causation—blood loss, injuries, excessive fats and sugars, frustration.

Common Health Issues—cough, cramps, dysentery, food poisoning, hemorrhage (excess bleeding), morning sickness, nausea, opiate addiction, vomiting, whooping cough.

IRIS VERSICOLOR
Iris Versicolor (Blue Flag)

KEYNOTES
VOMITING OF SOUR OR BITTER, MIGRAINE WITH VISION LOSS, PANCREATITIS.

SYMPTOMS
Physical symptoms—MIGRAINE over LEFT EYE with nausea, alternates sides. Sunday migraines. Gastric headache preceded by vision loss with sour, acrid vomiting of bile or acid, and copious urination. Greasy nose, tongue, gums. SALIVA while talking. Right shoulder pain. Vomiting after eating sweets. Vomiting roping mucus. STOMACH BURNS WITH SOUR TASTE. PANCREATITIS. Psoriasis of elbows, knees. SCIATICA, LEFT. Stool greasy. All symptoms better by the seashore. Body has an acidic odor.

Mental/Emotional symptoms—irritable. Laughs at self, easily frustrated. Alternating mood. Charming. Caretaker type. Restless at night. Depressive.

MODALITIES
Worse—periodically or weekly, spring, fall, mental exhaustion, hot weather. Better—gentle motion, cold applications. Time—worse 2 to 3 A.M., weekly, after midnight.

ASSOCIATED
Sides—LEFT.

Organs—pancreas, thyroid, GI tract, liver.

Gender—masculine or feminine.

Personalities—weekly headache of intellectual workers, artists.

Causation—not important.

Common Health Issues—headaches, migraines, nausea, pancreatitis, vomiting.

KALI ARS
Kali Arsenicosum (Potassium Arsenate)

KEYNOTES
PANIC ATTACKS, ANXIETY and FEAR with all problems, uses ANTI-ANXIETY DRUGS, Sleepless 1 to 3 A.M. with anxiety and fear.

SYMPTOMS
Physical symptoms—swollen lower eyelid (Kali carb for upper eyelids). Burning in throat. Edema (swelling). Vomiting after drinking cold water (Phosphorus). Backache with right sciatica. Eczema worse in warmth. COLD body. Anxious at night, worse 1 to 3 A.M. Worse with touch and noise.

Mental/Emotional symptoms—HEALTH FEARS (Arsenicum Album), especially in heart disease—must constantly check blood pressure. Fears of fainting. Must use anti-anxiety drugs. Superstitious. Claustrophobic. Speechless. INTROVERTED but desires company. Ritualistic behaviors. ANXIETY IN MID-CHEST.

MODALITIES
Worse—1 to 3 A.M., cold feet, touch, warmth of bed, lying down. Better—rainy days. Time—worse 1 to 3 A.M., asthma.

ASSOCIATED
Sides—right.

Organs—cardiovascular, nervous system, kidneys.

Gender—masculine or feminine.

Personalities—not important.

Causation—chronic anxiety.

Common Health Issues—allergies, anxiety, asthma, eczema, panic attacks, psoriasis.

KALI BICH
Kali Bichromicum (Potassium Bichromate)

KEYNOTES
THICK YELLOW-GREEN gluey MUCUS, craves BEER, SINUS INFECTION.

SYMPTOMS
Physical symptoms—aversion to light and noise. Headaches over eyebrows. Vision loss before headaches. MUCUS PROBLEMS, yellow-green ropey gluey discharges. Maxillary (cheek-jaw) SINUSITIS. Thirsty, craves BEER. Hair on tongue sensation. SWEATS on upper lip. Angina (heart pain). Heartburn after eating. Small stomach ulcers. Skin: THIRD DEGREE BURNS. LUPUS ERYTHEMATOSUS. Pains appear and disappear suddenly. Pains wander. PAIN IN SMALL SPOTS. Obesity. COLD body. Better or worse in heat.

Mental/Emotional symptoms—rigid rules and routines, wants regularity. Materialistic. Conformist. Impatient. Sadness better after eating. Talks to themselves.

MODALITIES
Worse—cold, mornings, waking, hot weather, beer, alcohol. Better—heat or cold weather, eating, vomiting, napping, motion. Time—worse 2 to 3 A.M., worse after sleeping.

ASSOCIATED
Sides—either, more right-sided.

Organs—stomach lining, mucus membranes, heart, joints.

Gender—masculine or feminine.

Personalities—bureaucrats, dancers, love fishing.

Causation—alcohol or beer intake.

Common Health Issues—arthritis, burns: third degree, headaches, lupus, migraines, mucus, nasal congestion, postnasal drip, sinusitis.

KALI BROM
Kali Bromatum (Potassium Bromide)

KEYNOTES
Fidgety fingers, wringing hands, scarring acne, religiosity versus sexual excesses.

SYMPTOMS
Physical symptoms—pale, drunk look, vacant, and expressionless face. Epilepsy followed by a headache, ASSOCIATED with sexual excess. Rolling movement of eyeballs. Stroke symptoms. ACNE on forehead of obese people. High blood pressure. Obesity. Psoriasis. Rashes in winter. Cysts. Lipomas (fatty tumors). Trembling. Nervous tapping or moving legs and hands. Staggering walk. Rectal polyps.

Mental/Emotional symptoms—hallucinations, feeling satanic or empowered by God. Morality vs. immorality. RELIGIOUS DELUSIONS (Veratrum Album). Despair of salvation. Suspicious, paranoid. Helpless, insecure. Forgetfulness, loses words. Crying and laughing fits. High sex drive. Childish behavior. Schizophrenia. Deep depression. Painful delusions and insomnia, especially in the elderly (Arsenicum Album, Calcarea Carb). Night terrors.

MODALITIES
Worse—thinking, emotions, excessive sex, puberty, hot weather, pregnancy, new moon. Better—being busy. Time—night worse, especially 2 A.M.; moaning, grinding teeth, sleepwalking.

ASSOCIATED
Sides—right.
Organs—nervous system, mind, genitalia, skin.
Gender—feminine.
Personalities—not important.
Causation—loss of business (Aurum metallicum), sexual excess, worry.
Common Health Issues—acne on forehead (main use), also acne back, shoulders, and chest with scarring in obese people, religious delusions as if evil or a servant of God, psoriasis, stroke symptoms.

KALI CARB
Kali Carbonicum (Potassium carbonate)

KEYNOTES
OBESITY, DUTY, WORSE DRAFTS and 2-4 A.M., GAS, WATER RETENTION ANKLES.

SYMPTOMS
Physical symptoms—haggard, gray complexion. Freckles on pale face. Upper eyelid swelling. Back problems. Spinal hot-poker pains from 2 until 4 A.M. Sweats on painful parts. OBESITY, especially in the elderly. Asthma, bronchitis, pneumonia, whooping cough. Craves sweets. Gas. Stomach ulcers. Arthritis—knees and hips. Stiff stitching pain. SWELLING in feet or ankles. Water retention. All symptoms WORSE DRAFTS.

Mental/Emotional symptoms—logical, self-assured, dogmatic, no compromise, rigid, exacting, anal-retentive, stoic, controlling. Fear of losing control. Duty. Holds emotions in stomach. Talks to themselves. Hoarding, possessive. Wants company not sympathy. Can't stand up for themselves. Polite and dignified. Averse to being touched. Startles easily, worse from noise. Mood-swings before menstruation.

MODALITIES
Worse—cold, fluid loss, physical exertion, sex, suppress menstruation. Better—open air, warmth, belching, dry warm weather, moving. Time worse—2 to 4 A.M. There is asthma or other hot poker pains.

ASSOCIATED
Sides—right.
Organs—heart, blood, kidneys, lungs, muscles, mucus membranes.
Gender—masculine or feminine.
Personalities—exacting—bookkeepers, treasurers, translators, attorneys, police, religious people.
Causation—NWS (never well since) pneumonia, skin eruption suppression in childhood from use of steroid creams.
Common Health Issues—asthma, backache, bronchitis, cough, eyelid swelling, leg-ankle swelling pleurisy, pneumonia.

KALI MUR
Kali Muriaticum (Potassium chloride)

KEYNOTES
Mucus congestion, white mucus, eustachian tube blockage.

SYMPTOMS
Physical symptoms—eustachian tube blockage. Cracking noises in ears. Frontal sinusitis. White mucus discharges. Tonsillitis. Respiratory mucus. Coughing. Pneumonia, coughing up white to grey mucus. Can't tolerate fatty foods. Joint swelling. Muscle cramps. Hemorrhoids. Medium fever of 101-103 degrees. Thirsty. Cold body.

Mental/Emotional symptoms—regular, down-to-earth. Quarrels with family. Provoked easily. Introvert. Aversion to noise. Wants to sit still. Foggy. Alternating moods.

MODALITIES
Worse—open air, heat of bed, dampness, cold drinks, motion, fatty foods. Better—rubbing, cold drinks. Time—worse night.

ASSOCIATED
Sides—left.
Organs—ears, throat, mucus membranes.
Gender—masculine or feminine.
Personalities—not important.
Causation—vaccination or injury.
Common Health Issues—allergies, mucus—white; ears, eustachian tubes, hemorrhoids, sinusitis.

KALI PHOS
Kali Phosphoricum (Potassium phosphate)

KEYNOTES
NERVOUS SYSTEM, NERVOUS IRRITABILITY, DEPRESSION.

SYMPTOMS
Physical symptoms—tinnitus, buzzing ears. Bad breath. Pale. Blushing. Yellow mucus discharges, bad odor. Nervous chattering teeth. Rings hands. Bad smelling vaginal discharges. Sexual excitement. Diarrhea bad smelling. Sensitive, irritable, easily startled. Weakness, exhaustion and decay. Sensitive to noise. Elderly people. Better by walking slowly.

Mental/Emotional symptoms—mental or physical exhaustion, everything seems like a task. Anxiety and nervous dread. Night terrors. Insomnia. Business cares. Sensitivity. Restless babies. Depression. Nervous irritability. Blushing.

MODALITIES
Worse—mental effort, physical exertion, anxiety, worry, cold, puberty, sex, touch, pain. Better—warmth, rest, gentle motion. Time—worse at night.

ASSOCIATED
Sides—one-sided.

Organs—nervous system.

Gender—masculine or feminine.

Personalities—business professionals, nursing mothers.

Causation—injuries, frustration, mental overwork.

Common Health Issues—depression, fatigue, insomnia, mental fog, nervous breakdown.

KALI SULPH
Kali Sulphuricum (Potassium sulphate)

KEYNOTES
SKIN, brown spots et cetera, HIGH FEVER, vitiligo (lack of skin pigmentation).

SYMPTOMS
Physicals symptoms—facial acne. Hates eggs, loves sweets. Yellow mucus discharges. Sweats easily. Rattling chest mucus, High fever of 103-105 degrees. Skin: VITILIGO (lack of pigmentation), brown spots (cholasma). Yellow scales. Cold hands and feet. Wandering joint pains. Warm-blooded person.

Mental/Emotional symptoms—lazy, impatient, worse consolation. Self-pity. Disgraced, insulted, nightmares, hurried, timid, confused, claustrophobia.

MODALITIES
Worse—warmth, noise, consolation, evening. Better—cool air, belching, passing gas. Time worse in evenings.

ASSOCIATED
Sides—both.

Organs—lungs, skin, glands, liver.

Gender—masculine or feminine.

Personalities—not important.

Causation—temperature extremes or injuries.

Common Health Issues—mucus, dandruff, eczema, psoriasis, sinusitis, vitiligo.

KREOSOTUM
Kreosotum (Beechwood Kreosote)

KEYNOTES
CORROSIVE VAGINAL DISCHARGES, OFFENSIVE DISCHARGES
ESPECIALLY MENSTRUATION, DECAY.

SYMPTOMS
Physical symptoms—vertigo: falling sensation. Tinnitus. Impaired
hearing. Teeth, premature decay (or black teeth, of first teeth in children). Gums painful and swollen. OBESITY. Bleeding from small
wounds. Burning, offensive smelling discharges. Bedwetting. Painful
menstruation with heavy bleeding. Vaginal discharges burning, yellow
staining. Pain the day after sex. Irritating, burning diarrhea. Old wom-
en. Menopause symptoms.

Mental/Emotional symptoms—claims wellness in sickness. Headstrong.
Introvert. Thoughts vanish. Dissatisfied with everything, cross, obsti-
nate, throws things when angry. Emotions cause physical pulsations.
Fears and dreams of rape. Fears sex.

MODALITIES
Worse—teething in children, rest, cold, pregnancy, menstruation,
touch, standing. Better—sitting, warmth, hot foods, motion, sneezing.
Time—worse from 6 P.M. to 6 A.M.

ASSOCIATED
Sides—left.

Organs—gastrointestinal tract, gums, teeth, female genitalia, mucus
membranes.

Gender—feminine.

Personalities—not important.

Causations—not important.

Common Health Issues—blood poisoning, cholera infantum, digestive
ulcers, gangrene, hoarseness, putrid odor, tooth decay, irritating vaginal
discharge.

LAC CANINUM
Lac Caninum (Dog's milk)

KEYNOTES
ALTERNATES SIDES, WORSE TOUCH, ALTERNATING MOODS, BREASTS, wandering pains.

SYMPTOMS
Physical symptoms—headaches alternate sides. Photophobia. Earwax—black. Green discharges, odorless. Vertigo as if floating. Tonsillitis, glazed appearance. Low blood pressure. Breasts swollen before menstruation. Mastitis on least movement. Dries up milk in lactating women. Skin ulcers that appear shiny. Sciatica right side. Wandering or crosswise arthritis (upper right to lower left, etc.). Easy sexual excitement. Can't stand to be touched. Alternating sides. Warm blooded. Everything better hard pressure.

Mental/Emotional symptoms—unsettled, anxious, nervous, startled easily. Cries easily. Absent-minded. Hypersensitive. Low self-esteem, self-loathing. Aggressive, angry. Fears fainting. Fears insects and ghosts. Compelled to wash hands. Loves dogs. Despondent. Alternating moods.

MODALITIES
Worse—touch, jarring, pressure, empty swallowing, menstruation, resting. Better—cold, cold drinks, open-air. Time—worse one morning, next the evening, worse at night.

ASSOCIATED
Sides—alternating.

Organs—throat, female sex organs, nerves, breasts.

Gender—feminine.

Personalities—not important.

Causation—diphtheria.

Common Health Issues—diphtheria, painful breasts, delusions, migraines, tonsillitis.

LACHESIS
Lachesis muta (Bushmaster snake)

KEYNOTES
TALKATIVE, CONSTRICTED THROAT, BIPOLAR, worse waking.

SYMPTOMS
Physical symptoms—Purplish or bluish skin. Doesn't want anything tight, especially around neck. Talkative. Trembling tongue. LISPING. Salivation when talking. CONSTRICTED THROAT. Appendicitis. Never well since menopause. sometimes red hair, freckles, mostly large chested, low-cut dresses. Throbbing pains.

Mental/Emotional symptoms—mostly EXTROVERTED. Intense. Wants to be admired. Fashionable. Mind is active at night. Talkative, jumps from one subject to another. Witty, satire. Opinionated, quarrelsome, self-centered, arrogant. Claustrophobic. ALCOHOLISM. Religious fanaticism. Suspicious, paranoid. JEALOUS. Often BIPOLAR. High sex drive.

MODALITIES
Worse—waking, heat, swallowing, pressure, sexual climax, alcohol, temperature extremes. Better—open air, urination, menstruation, cold drinks, hard pressure. Time—worse on waking.

ASSOCIATED
Sides—LEFT. Or left to right.

Organs—nervous system, throat, female organs, circulation, liver.

Gender—FEMININE.

Personalities—high society, sales, teachers, nuns.

Causation—sleep loss, emotions, masturbation, menopause, alcoholism.

Common Health Issues—alcoholism, bedsores, bipolar, boils, digestive ulcers, heart disorders, high blood pressure, mania, menopause, schizophrenia, wounds.

LACTIC ACID
Lacticum Acidum (Lactic acid)

KEYNOTES
DIABETES, morning sickness, nausea, excessive fluids or lacking fluids.

SYMPTOMS
Physical symptoms—Excessive saliva, tastes salty. Hoarseness. Milk craving, or an aversion to milk. Emaciation with a large appetite—MUST EAT. Morning sickness. Nausea upon waking._Nausea in those with poor diet. Copious sweating with sour smell. Enlarged armpit glands. Weak limbs. Breast sensitive, tender, lactation profuse. Hypoglycemia. Diabetes with arthritis. Frequent copious urination, especially at night. Anemic, pale women who are depressive.

Mental/Emotional symptoms—irritable, complaining, sarcastic. Confused, forgetful. Overly organized. Discouraged when pregnant. Dreams of sex.

MODALITIES
Worse—smoking aggravates all symptoms. Time—restless at night.

ASSOCIATED
Sides—either.

Organs—digestion, muscles, joints, bone.

Gender—feminine.

Personalities—not important.

Causation—smoking.

Common Health Issues—aching pains, breast problems, diabetes, lymphatic gland enlargement, morning sickness, nausea.

LEDUM
Ledum Palustre (Marsh tea-wild rosemary)

KEYNOTES
WOUNDS, BRUISED PAIN, PUNCTURE WOUNDS, INSECT BITES OR STINGS.

SYMPTOMS
Physical symptoms—black eye. Nightly sweating. Gouty arthritis. Bruised sensation. Insect bites, itching worse in heat of bed. Puncture wounds. Used to prevent tetanus. Bruising. Poor wound healing. Anal deep-skin cracks. Ankles. Tendons. Stout muscular build. Feeling drunk. Feels cold.

Mental/Emotional symptoms—averse to people, loner. Hatred of human beings, hating, vengeful. Sadness. Confusion. Alcoholism.

MODALITIES
Worse—warmth, alcohol, injuries, motion, night. Better—cold, in ice water, resting. Time—worse at night.

ASSOCIATED
Sides—left upper and right lower.

Organs—joints, tendons, skin, periosteum, blood, nerves.

Gender—masculine or feminine.

Personalities—athletes.

Causation—injuries, bites, stings, puncture wounds.

Common Health Issues—anal deep-skin cracks, bites, black eyes, bruising, puncture wounds, poison ivy, vaccinations, wounds.

LILIUM TIG
Lilium Tigrinum (Tiger Lily)

KEYNOTES
FEMALE COMPLAINTS, WILD THOUGHTS, HEART PROBLEMS, hysterical rage.

SYMPTOMS
Physical symptoms—nearsighted. Great appetite, easily satiated. Sensation as if sharp pain through left nipple to heart. Left breast. Heart feels as if grasped, palpitations, fluttering. Burning palms of hands and soles of the feet. Strong sexuality. Menstruation stops when lying down. Uterine prolapse, uterus feels like it's falling out. Left ovary. Desires open air. Pains radiates. Burning pains. Pressing pains. Pains in small spots.

Mental/Emotional symptoms—arrogant, self-important, ungrateful, offended easily. Hates consolation. Has a crazy feeling in the head. Timid. Often unmarried women. Fears of incurable diseases. Must keep busy to distract from sexual feelings. Sex versus religious values, feels doomed of salvation. Curses.

MODALITIES
Worse warmth, consolation, walking, after menstruation. Better—cool air, keeping busy, sunset, pressure, crossing legs, sitting. Time—worse at night.

ASSOCIATED
Sides—left.

Organs—circulation, female genitals, heart, nerves.

Gender—feminine.

Personalities—not important.

Causation—celibacy or sexual excess, childbirth, menopause.

Common Health Issues—astigmatism, depression, heart disorders, ovary problems, uterine problems, uterine prolapse.

LOBELIA
Lobelia Inflata (Indian Tobacco)

KEYNOTES
NAUSEA, VOMITING with conditions, sensitive to TOBACCO.

SYMPTOMS
Physical symptoms—metallic taste in mouth with excess salivation. Feels better with beer. Heart feels as if it would stand still. MUSCLE SPASMS. Spasmodic asthma with stomach weakness. Prickling sensation. Weak lungs. COLD SWEAT. Obesity. STOMACH feels faint. Nausea with salivation, prickling sensation, cold sweat, exhaustion, and pain. Cold body. Aversion or allergy to tobacco.

Mental/Emotional symptoms—health fears. Hysteria. Lump in throat. Breathing issues from emotions. Overly organized. Fears of heart disease and predicts death.

MODALITIES
Worse—sleep, tobacco, touch, motion. Better—eating, warmth. Time—not important.

ASSOCIATED
Sides—either.

Gender—masculine or feminine.

Organs—respiratory, nerves, heart, secretions.

Personalities—not important.

Causation—alcoholism, drug addictions, smoking habit.

Common Health Issues—asthma, heartburn, nausea, tobacco habit effects, vomiting.

LYCOPODIUM
Lycopodium Clavatum (Club moss)

KEYNOTES
WORSE FROM 4-8 P.M., INFERIORITY COMPLEX, LIVER PROBLEMS, NOISY GAS.

SYMPTOMS
Physical symptoms—old-looking face, wrinkled forehead—horizontal lines. Haughty look. Arcus senilis (stress ring of opacity on ring of cornea). Dystonia-deafness. Cold right ear. Allergies hay fever, nostrils flare to catch breath. Larynx (voicebox) moves up and down. Vomiting undigested food. Noisy GAS. Water retention of lower body. Puberty delayed. Carpal tunnel syndrome. LEAN person. Intellectual. Weaker upper body. Poor physicality. DRYNESS.

Mental/Emotional symptoms—the "little dictator," kissing up to superiors, but abusive to perceived inferiors. Lack of confidence, poor self-esteem. Inflated ego. Helplessness. Fears responsibility. Irritable on waking. Keen intellect. Indecision. Writer's block. Males flirt. Boasting.

MODALITIES
Worse—waking, wind, pressure of clothes, indigestion, lying on the right side, bread. Better—motion, belching, urinating, open air. Time—worse from 4-8 P.M., and 3-4 A.M.

ASSOCIATED
Sides—right, or right to left.

Organs—liver, GI tract, urinary, longs.

Gender—masculine or feminine.

Personalities—police, politics, business people.

Causation—emotional fright, ailments from sugar, sweets or wine.

Common Health Issues—aneurysm, belching, bloating, colitis, diabetes, dyslexia, gas, hemorrhoids, hepatitis, hypoglycemia, sciatica, stage fright.

MAG CARB
Magnesia Carbonica* (Magnesium carbonate)

KEYNOTES
SOUR everything, attitude, smells etc., worse DAIRY, craves meat.

SYMPTOMS
Physical symptoms—hyperthyroid (overactive thyroid). Desires meat. Sour smell. Poor muscle power. Obesity. Worn out. Flabby. Gassy. Chilly, pain with sweating. Weeping during pregnancy. Green diarrhea. Adults—reserved, tendency to nervous breakdown. Children—were abandoned, sensitive, nervous, poor muscle power with tendency to bronchitis. Stuttering. Babies—colic, milk passes undigested, sour smell, teething, irritable and cry easily. Sensitivity to touch. All symptoms WORSE MILK.

Mental/Emotional symptoms—sour temperament, oversensitive. Peacemaker, avoids conflict. Feels unloved by friends, parents. Insecure, emotional instability. Children—problems with reading, and especially writing. Hyperactive. Fear something bad will happen.

MODALITIES
Worse—night, noise, change of weather, cold, milk, slight touch, before and during menstruation, pregnancy, warmth of bed. Better—motion, open air, after menstruation, after stool, walking. Time—worse at night.

ASSOCIATED
Sides—left.

Organs—digestive tract, nervous system.

Gender—feminine, women and girls.

Personalities—not important.

Causation—emotional trauma, injuries, poor nutrition.

Common Health Issues—belching, colic, dairy allergies, diarrhea, failure to thrive, heartburn, insomnia, malnutrition, vaginal discharges.

*Not in found in Conditions chapter.

MAG MUR
Magnesia Muriatica* (Magnesium chloride)

KEYNOTES
MILK AGGRAVATES, PACIFISTS, SMALL INTESTINE, digestive disturbances.

SYMPTOMS
Physical symptoms—sour expression on face. Wrinkled forehead. Vertical cracks near root of nose. Hyperventilation. Carpal tunnel syndrome. Ganglion cysts. Warts. Chronic indigestion from small intestine problems. Liver problems, easily frightened. Women with spasms, hysteria, and uterine problems. Children suffer with fighting parents. Waking up tired. Everything is worse with milk.

Mental/Emotional symptoms—extroverted. Mild. Disconnected. Nervous. Excitable. Pacifism. Anxious and hurried. They are responsible, live for service and sacrifice. Depression. Dislike confrontations.

MODALITIES
Worse—milk, lying on the right side, eating, salt, closing the eyes. Better—hard pressure, limbs hanging down, cool open-air, gentle motion. Time—worse at night.

ASSOCIATED
Sides—right.

Organs—adrenals, liver, nervous system, small intestine.

Gender—feminine.

Personalities—pacifists.

Causation—anger, frustration, sexual excesses.

Common Health Issues—cirrhosis of liver, constipation, dairy allergies, diarrhea, heart palpitations, hepatitis, liver disorders, menstrual pain, nerve disorders.

*Not in found in Conditions chapter.

MAG PHOS
Magnesia Phosphorica (Magnesium phosphate)

KEYNOTES
CRAMPS (mostly right-sided), shooting pains.

SYMPTOMS
Physical symptoms—right-sided, facial, nerve pain, wakes from pains. Teething children. Makes strange gestures. Radiating pain, spasms, or cramping pains better when doubling over and applying warmth and pressure, worse touch. Shooting or radiating or electrical pains. Pain causes exhaustion, restlessness. Phantom limb pains. Sciatica, right side. Nervous young people, or tired or exhausted persons. Everything WORSE WITH COLD.

Mental/Emotional symptoms—extrovert, impulsive, artistic, intellectual. Nervous, restless, intense, talks about pains. Fears the dark, being touched, and thunderstorms. Bad dreams. Over sensitive to pain, noise, and excitement. Willful.

MODALITIES
Worse—cold, touch, night, motion. Better—warmth everything, pressure, doubling over, rubbing. Time—worse at night, worse from 4 to 8 P.M. (Lycopodium).

ASSOCIATED
Sides—right.

Organs—nervous system, heart.

Personalities—musicians, carpenters, sewing.

Causation—emotions, muscle overuse, cold exposure.

Common Health Issues—angina (heart pain), cramps, painful menstruation, facial nerve pains (neuralgia), rib pain, paralysis, sciatica, toothaches.

MERCURY CORROSIVE
Mercurius Corrosivus (Mercuris chloride)

KEYNOTES
INFECTIONS, severe diarrhea or dysentery, UTIs with burning and bloody discharge, EXCESS SALIVA.

SYMPTOMS
Physical symptoms—vertigo and deafness. Burning sore eyes. Ulcerative canker sores. Thirsty, with bad smelling saliva. Desires cold drinks. Irritating discharges. Mucus membranes dark red. Cold. Sweating. Sweating at night. Acute kidney damage with burning pains. Burning pains. Tightening sensation. UTIs (urinary tract infections). Urethritis. Hot urine, passes drop by drop. Urgency to stool but little release.

Mental/Emotional symptoms—instability. Closed, disconnected. Conservative. Anxiety trying to sleep. Rocking. Mind sluggish with poor digestion.

MODALITIES
Worse—after urination, stool, swallowing, fats, sex, motion, autumn, hot days and cool nights, dysentery. Better—resting. Time—worse at night.

ASSOCIATED
Sides—left.

Organs—throat, glands, bladder, kidneys.

Gender—masculine or feminine.

Personalities—not important.

Causation—suppressed gonorrhea from antibiotics.

Common Health Issues—bladder problems, burning pains, digestive ulcers, dysentery, gonorrhea, iritis, kidney problems, severe diarrhea, urinary tract infection (UTI).

MERCURY SOL
Mercurius Solubis—akin to Mecurius Vivus (Quicksilver)

KEYNOTES
Infections, yellow-green discharges, temperature sensitive, emotional extremes, metallic taste or smell.

SYMPTOMS
Physical symptoms—excess salivation. Any yellow-greenish pus discharges. Sensitive to draft. Narrow temperature-comfort range. Tremors. Boils. Pus. Unusual symptoms—milk in breasts on boys or girls.

Mental/Emotional symptoms—the "Mad Hatter," depression, anxiety, irrational fears, avoids people. Shallow personality—goes from one relationship, or one job, to another.

MODALITIES
Worse—night, sweating, heat, drafts, discharges. Better—narrow temperature range, mornings, rest. Time—worse 3-4 P.M. with low energy, better 11 P.M., waking, and at 5 A.M.

ASSOCIATED
Sides—left, but either.

Organs—mucus membranes, liver, kidney, spine, joints, salivary glands, lymphatic system, genitals.

Gender—masculine or feminine.

Personalities—police versus criminals (Al Capone), lawyers, judges, journalists.

Causation—fright, sweat, gonorrhea suppressed from antibiotic use.

Common Health Issues—food allergies, canker sores, mononucleosis, multiple sclerosis, Parkinson's with tremors.

MEZEREUM
Mezereum (Spurge olive)

KEYNOTES
SKIN ERUPTIONS, yellow, oozing, gluey scabs with pus underneath.
SHINGLES on chest, post shingles pain.

SYMPTOMS
Physical symptoms—curly hair. Dandruff with thick crust with pus.
Whiplash. Excess salivation. Desires fat. Gastritis—stomach ulcers.
Shingles, especially on the chest. Sudden pains. Burning pains worse
with light touch. Vaccination eruptions. Gout. Eczema. SKIN eruptions
which are oozy, gluey, and have thick crust with pus underneath. Severe
itching. Testes enlarged, PAINLESS scrotum enlargement. Coccyx
injury(tailbone).

Mental/Emotional symptoms—anger at trifle, says mean things but is
soon sorry. Averse to being touched. Religious and financial depression. Anxiety from stomach, everything feels empty. Apathetic, staring. Frustrated, irresolute. Hypochondriac. Disoriented. Vanishing of
thoughts while speaking.

MODALITIES
Worse—night, warmth of bed, vaccinations, cold air, draft, motion,
touch, cold washing. Better—eating, stooping, wrapping up, open air,
milk. Time—worse at night.

ASSOCIATED
Sides—left.

Organs—stomach, nerves, skin.

Gender—masculine or feminine.

Personalities—not important.

Causation—suppressed eczema, vaccinations.

Common Health Issues—eczema, eruptions, itching, neuralgia, shingles, skin problems, testicles enlarged.

MURIATIC ACID
Muriaticum acidum (Hydrochloric acid)

KEYNOTES
exhaustion, introverted, VERTIGO, INVOLUNTARY STOOLS.

SYMPTOMS
Physical symptoms—vertigo with nausea. Cankers with salivation. Can't stand meat. Heart palpitations felt in face. FEVERS. Liver problems. Burning sensation. Muscle weakness. Weakness. DEBILITY. Sores. Hemorrhoids during pregnancy. Stools difficult. Involuntary stools, urinating while passing stools. DIARRHEA. Worse lying on right side, better turning to the left side.

Mental/Emotional symptoms—introverted, suffers in silence. Never self-satisfied. Muttering and moaning, finds no pleasure in life. Exhausted easily from work.

MODALITIES
Worse—wet weather, walking, cold drinks, touch, sweating, after sleep, menstruation, urinating. Better—motion, warm, lying on left side. Time—worse at 11 P.M.

ASSOCIATED
Sides—left.

Organs—blood, muscle, mucus membranes, tongue, heart, mouth.

Gender—masculine or feminine.

Personalities—drug addicts.

Causation—depletion from alcohol or other drug addictions.

Common Health Issues—alcoholism, bedsores, digestive ulcers, drug addictions, fevers, hemorrhoids, typhoid fever.

NAT MUR
Natrum Muriaticum (Sodium chloride)

KEYNOTES
WATER BALANCE, DRYNESS, chronic GRIEF, INTROVERT, craves salt.

SYMPTOMS
Physical symptoms—greasy around hairline. Crave salt. Dryness. Tendency to Herpes 1 and 2. Menopause—vaginal dryness, aversion to sex. Lean, thin person. All symptoms worse or better by the seashore.

Mental/Emotional symptoms—introvert, holds emotions inside, cries in private. Hates sympathy. Easily hurt but doesn't show it publicly. Feels responsible. Defensive. Female often doesn't marry or remarry after a bad divorce. Loves to read.

MODALITIES
Worse—sunrise, heat, sun, sympathy, puberty, seashore, crying. Better—cool, sweating, rest, regular meals. Time—all symptoms worse from 9 to 11 A.M.

ASSOCIATED
Sides—left.

Organs—blood, fluids, mucus membranes.

Gender—masculine or feminine.

Personalities—counselors.

Causation—grief, betrayal, disappointed love, head injury, sun exposure.

Common Health Issues—allergies hay fever, autism, depression, herpes 1 and 2, high blood pressure, impotence, infertility, sunstroke, vaginitis.

NAT PHOS
Natrum Phosphoricum* (Sodium phosphate)

KEYNOTES
body acid-balance, heartburn, yellow discharges, parasites.

SYMPTOMS
Physical symptoms—eyes: one pupil dilated, squinting. Yellow coating inside mouth. Sour belching. Crave sour, fried foods. Excess stomach acid (heartburn). Excess lactic acid in muscles and joints. Gouty arthritis. Yellow or creamy discharges. Insect bites. Kidney stones. Intestinal worms in children with colic and grinding teeth. Noisy gas. Ankle eczema.

Mental/Emotional symptoms—reserved, apprehensive, INTROVERTED. Fearful, fear of dogs, easily startled. Apathy to loved ones.

MODALITIES
Worse—SUGAR, DAIRY, storms, drafts, night. Better—pressure, cold open air. Time—worse nights.

ASSOCIATED
Sides—either.

Organs—nervous system, blood, digestive, genitals.

Gender—masculine or feminine.

Personalities—not important.

Causation—poor diet, alcohol.

Common Health Issues—acidity, diarrhea, digestive ulcers, gas, heartburn, hives, jaundice, vaginitis, worms.

*Not in found in Conditions chapter.

NAT SULPH
Natrum Sulphuricum (Sodium sulphate)

KEYNOTES
traumatic head injury, water regulator, Asthma, especially from cold humid conditions, rattling in chest 4 to 5 A.M. LIVER issues-yellow discharges.

SYMPTOMS
Physical symptoms—head injury, which may progress to epilepsy, to blindness, to suicide. Never well since change of personality and life-style from head injury Yellow discharges. Warm blooded but feels cold. Gallbladder stones. Enlarged liver, hepatitis. GLUTEN INTOLERANCE (Carcinosin or Iodium). Sciatica, right sided.

Mental/Emotional symptoms—sensitive to noise, depression, suicidal, epileptic—all after head injury. Closed. Objective. Very responsible individuals. Spiritual, duty to God. Not a morning person. Avoids conflict. Alternating moods. Not very emotional. Music can cause emotions.

MODALITIES
Worse—dampness, head injuries, lifting, touch, pressure, springtime (dampness). Better—warm, hot, dry weather, changing positions, sitting up, after breakfast. Time—worse from 2 to 5 A.M.

ASSOCIATED
Sides—right.

Organs—liver, pancreas, head, brain.

Gender—masculine or feminine.

Personalities—business people, religious orders.

Causation—traumatic head injury, living in cold damp house.

Common Health Issues—asthma, concussion, depression, epilepsy, head injury, hepatitis, liver problems, suicidal, photophobia, meningitis.

NITRIC ACID
Nitricum Acididum (Nitric acid)

KEYNOTES
WORSE TOUCH, SPLINTER PAINS, ANAL DEEP-SKIN CRACKS, worse ANTIBIOTICS.

SYMPTOMS
Physical symptoms—pale sunken face, old people. Severe acne. Cracked tongue. Weakness. Emaciation. Nosebleeds with chest problems, worse when crying. Reddish brown spots on skin. Crusts, deep skin cracks (fissures). PAINS SPLINTER-LIKE. Bad-smelling discharges. Strong urine odor. ANAL FISSURES (deep skin cracks). Diarrhea. Lean persons. Chilly person. Angry when touched.

Mental/Emotional symptoms—selfish. Fears of death and health issues, anxious about health. Resentful, bitter, won't accept apologies. Aggressive tone, manipulative, angry about own mistakes. Revengeful, bad temper, cursing, vindictive, pessimistic—holds grudges. Easily offended.

MODALITIES
Worse—touch, jarring, motion, cold, sweating, change of weather or temperature, being awake at night, WAKING. Better—good weather, steady pressure, warmth, rides in cars. Time—worse at night.

ASSOCIATED
Sides—left.

Organs—mouth, anus, mucus membranes, lymphatics, prostate, liver.

Gender—masculine or feminine.

Personalities—actors, singers with laryngitis or hoarseness.

Causation—sleep loss, caretaking others, antibiotics.

Common Health Issues—antibiotics, anal deep-skin cracks, diarrhea, digestive ulcers, emaciation, hemorrhages (excess bleeding), hemorrhoids, proctitis, ringworm, spinal injury, syphilis, tuberculosis, warts.

NUX VOMICA
Nux Vomica (Poison nut)

KEYNOTES
SEDENTARY, STIMULANTS, IRRITABLE, MALE, passive-aggressive.

SYMPTOMS
Physical symptoms—sensitive to noise, odors, light, touch, music. TIAs (strokes). Craves stimulants. Tired after eating. Gastritis—food sits as if rock in stomach. Sedentary lifestyle. Constipation. Hemorrhoids. Parasites. Cardiovascular problems from bad diet. Worse loss of sleep, waking 3 A.M. (the "liver hour" in Chinese medicine). Physically strong, muscular.

Mental/Emotional symptoms—extrovert. Lack of respect, interrupting. Zealous and fiery temperament, ambitious, driven to accomplish goals. Irritable to violent. Impatient, competitive. Fight fault-finding, jealous, quarrelsome. Fears of commitment. High sex drive. Overly organized.

MODALITIES
Worse—cold, draft, stimulants, being sedentary, overeating, mental fatigue, noise. Better—urination, rest, hot drinks, milk, loosening clothes, passing gas, warmth. Time—worse 3 to 4 A.M.

ASSOCIATED
Sides—RIGHT.

Organs—LIVER, GI tract, nervous system, urinary, respiratory.

Gender—MASCULINE.

Personalities—workaholics, managers, high-level business people, sales.

Causation—laxative abuse, alcohol, drug abuse, tobacco, prescription medications.

Common Health Issues—delirium tremens, drug addiction, heartburn, hangovers, hemorrhoids, liver disorders, morning sickness, nausea, photophobia, stomach disorders.

OPIUM
Papaver Somniferum* (Poppy)

KEYNOTES
STUPOR, COMA, SEVERE CONSTIPATION, LACK OF PAIN.

SYMPTOMS
Physical symptoms—dull. Euphoric. Drunken appearance. Head injury—sleepy—coma—pupils non-reactive. Face dark red. Sweaty skin. Breathing uneven. Picks at clothes. Makes gestures. Strange body positions. Constipation—paralysis of muscles, hard black balls. Involuntary stools from fright. Lack of pain—just wants to sleep. Sleepwalking with jerking, eyes or mouth open.

Mental/Emotional symptoms—fright. PTSD (post-traumatic stress disorder). Shame, reproach, wants to withdraw, not a fighter—no willpower. Nothing seems to faze them, shut down. Pleasant staring off into space or stupor. Poor judgment—rash, bold, fearless. Lies.

MODALITIES
Worse—emotions, alcohol, heat, sleep, stimulants, cold, sweating. Better—continuous walking, cold, open air. Time—worse sleeping.

ASSOCIATED
Sides—left.

Organs—nervous system, mind.

Gender—masculine or feminine.

Personalities—not important.

Causation—near-death experience, fright, alcohol, rape, carbon monoxide poisoning.

Common Health Issues—coma, delirium tremens, fear, meningitis, paralysis, PTSD (post-traumatic stress disorder), shock, strokes, trauma, vertigo.

*Not in found in Conditions chapter.

PETROLEUM
Oleum petrae (Crude rock oil)

KEYNOTES
DEEP, BLOODY SKIN CRACKS, WORSE WINTER, MOTION SICKNESS.

SYMPTOMS
Physical symptoms—vertigo on rising. Increased appetite, better eating. Hates fatty foods. Motion sickness. Foul armpits, smelly body odor. DRYNESS, increased discharges. Dirty deep cracks; hard, rough, thickened skin. Deep, bloody cracks, hands, fingers tips, folds of skin that are worse in winter. Thick greenish crust, burning, itching, redness, bleeding. Diarrhea. Cold in spots. All symptoms WORSE IN WINTER.

Mental/Emotional symptoms—quarrelsome, excitable, offended, frustrated, and confused. Abusive when drunk. Depression makes vision worse.

MODALITIES
Worse—motion, winter, eating, frustration, mental effort. Better in warm dry weather, lying with head high, summer. Time—worse during daytime.

ASSOCIATED
Sides—left.

Organs—skin, nervous system, mucus membranes, lungs, stomach.

Gender—masculine or feminine.

Personalities—machinists, exposure to toxicity, or petroleum products.

Causation—motion sickness, petroleum toxicity, suppressed skin conditions from use of steroid creams.

Common Health Issues—eczema, herpes, motion sickness, nausea, psoriasis, seasickness, skin cracks, skin problems, vertigo.

PHOSPHORICUM ACIDUM
Phosphoricum Acidum (Phosphoric acid)

KEYNOTES
BURNED OUT PHYSICALLY, EMOTIONALLY. CHRONIC FATIGUE,
GRIEF.

SYMPTOMS
Physical symptoms—gray hair early. Hair falls out with grief. Feels a
heavy weight on top of head. Pale sickly appearance. Sunken eyes, blue
circles under. Yellow spots in whites of eyes. Loss of appetite from grief.
Craves refreshing things. Dehydration. Emaciation from grief. Chronic
fatigue. Joints and muscles sweating. Ganglion cysts. Fingertips peeling.
Sciatica right-sided. Chilly body.

Mental/Emotional symptoms—mild, dreamy. Emotionally spent,
burnt out, apathy. Indifferent, doesn't like people, doesn't want to be
disturbed. Slow to grasp ideas. GRIEF, DISAPPOINTED LOVE. Life
changes. Often homesick, overwhelmed. Children grow too fast, with
weeping nightmares, bedwetting, frowning pains.

MODALITIES
Worse—fluid loss, emotions, cold, drafts, talking, masturbation, mental
activity, noise. Better—warmth, motion, pressure, naps, passing stool.
Time—not important.

ASSOCIATED
Sides—right.
Organs—nervous system, genitals, bones.
Gender—masculine or feminine.
Personalities—business persons who have lost their jobs, retirees.
Causation—growing too rapidly, fluid loss, sexual excess, over study,
drug abuse.
Common Health Issues—canker sores, diabetes, diarrhea, chronic fatigue, grief, homesickness, masturbation, weakness.

PHOSPHORUS
Phosphorus (element Phosphorus)

KEYNOTES
hemorrhages (excess bleeding) bright red BLOOD, SENSITIVE to others' energy, BURNING PAINS, FATTY LIVER.

SYMPTOMS
Physical symptoms—eye problems: retinitis, retinal detachment. Thirsty. Nosebleeds. Pancreas, hypoglycemic. Pneumonia with wings of nose flaring, can't breathe. Easily exhausted. BURNING PAINS. Hemorrhages (excess bleeding) of BRIGHT RED BLOOD. Relaxed open anus. Corns on heels. Chilly body. fidgety, generally tall, slender, fair skin, blond or red hair. Lightning victim. Antidotes anesthesia.

Mental/Emotional symptoms—EXTROVERT. Intelligent. Friendly, sympathetic, sensitive to others' energy, psychic, affectionate. Psychiatric patients. Impressionable, clairvoyant, and distracted. Suggestible, fears of dark and ghosts. Self-centered, scattered, spacey.

MODALITIES
Worse—emotions of others, cold, warm food, weather changes, mental fatigue. Better—sleep, eating, sitting up, lying on the right side, in the dark. Time—worse morning and evening.

ASSOCIATED
Sides—LEFT.

Organs—LUNGS, mucus membranes, nerves, blood vessels, GI tract.

Gender—masculine or feminine.

Personalities—artists, healers, psychics, priests, teachers, politicians, entertainers.

Causation—electroshock therapy, electrocution.

Common Health Issues—bronchitis, diabetes, hemophilia (bleeds easily), jaundice, liver problems, nosebleeds, pancreas, pneumonia, rickets.

PHYTOLACCA DEC
Phytolacca Decandra (Pokeweed, Pokeroot)

KEYNOTES
SWOLLEN GLANDS, SORE THROAT, MASTITIS.

SYMPTOMS
Physical symptoms—glands swollen and hard. Sinusitis, dark red tonsils, sore throat—especially left side with shooting pain into ears from swallowing. Excess mucus. Mumps. Weakness, exhaustion, stiffness. Feels sore. Has wandering pains (sharp). Boils. Mastitis—breasts swollen, hard, and tender—worse when nursing. Cracked nipples, chronic discharges. Worse cold damp wet.

Mental/Emotional symptoms—apathy about their appearance.

MODALITIES
Worse—motion, swallowing, weather changes, nursing, wet weather. Better—lying on stomach, rest, warm, dry weather, cold drinks. Time—pains worse night.

ASSOCIATED
Sides—right.

Organs—breasts, throat, back, kidneys, neck, digestive tract.

Gender—masculine or feminine.

Personalities—not important.

Causation—severe emotions, grief, injury, exposure to damp weather.

Common Health Issues—arthritis, boils, mastitis, breast problems, breastfeeding, glandular swelling, mumps, tonsillitis.

PICRIC ACID
Picricum Acidum (Picric Acid)

KEYNOTES
MENTAL AND PHYSICAL EXHAUSTION, TEST FUNK, SEXUAL excitement, poor function.

SYMPTOMS
Physical symptoms—ailments from mental work. Dilated pupils with headaches. Severe anemia (pernicious). Jaundice. Sensitive to heat. Skin conditions. Heaviness worse from physical motion. Burning pains. Male sexual excitement but loses erection easily. Impotence. Prostate enlargement (BPH) with male urine stoppage. Worn out mentally and physically. All symptoms worse in cold air.

Mental/Emotional symptoms—mental exhaustion, apathy, no willpower. Dreads taking tests—test funk, anxiety, confusion. Problems from grief and depression. Sexual thoughts.

MODALITIES
Worse—motion, mental effort or physical exertion, heat, study, wet hot weather, sperm loss, sexual excitement. Better—bandaging, sun, rest, cold air, water, rest. Time—not important.

ASSOCIATED
Sides—either.

Organs—nerves, kidneys, genitals.

Gender—masculine or feminine.

Personalities—mental-health workers.

Causation—mental overwork, emotional trauma.

Common Health Issues—boils, brain fog, debility, headaches, kidney problems, memory weakness, nervous exhaustion, urinary problems.

Podophyllum

PODOPHYLLUM
Podophyllum Pelatum (May-apple)

KEYNOTES
DIARRHEA yellow, PROLAPSE.

SYMPTOMS
Physical symptoms—sweating on scalp while sleeping. Headache with diarrhea. Loss of taste. Clenched jaws. Sweats with pain. Rubs liver region. Stomach pain, weakness. Gallstones. Abdominal weakness. Gurgling bowels. Pregnancy—swollen bluish labia. Prolapsed uterus, anus, rectum. Hemorrhoids from portal vein congestion. Offensive diarrhea, gas—explosive. Sleep—moaning, grinding teeth, lies on abdomen. All symptoms worse in summer.

Mental/Emotional symptoms—Delirious or talkative during fever. Thinks they will die. Depression with gastric issues.

MODALITIES
Worse—EARLY MORNING, eating, hot weather, teething, drinking, motion, bathing, over-straining muscles, stool. Better—rubbing liver, lying on abdomen, evening, bending forward. Time—worse 2 to 4 A.M., worse 4 to 5 A.M. with diarrhea.

ASSOCIATED
Sides—right.
Organs—LIVER, gallbladder, small intestines, rectum.
Gender—masculine or feminine.
Personalities—business people with mental fatigue.
Causation—LIVER problems.
Common Health Issues—diarrhea, yellow diarrhea, parasites, teething, uterus prolapse.

PULSATILLA
Pulsatilla Nigricans (Pasque-flower)

KEYNOTES
WEEPY, PEOPLE PLEASER, WANDERING SYMPTOMS, FEARS OF ABANDONMENT.

SYMPTOMS
Physical symptoms—pale face. Chronic sinusitis. Mucus discharge is bland, yellow greenish. HEAT INTOLERANCE. NO THIRST. Intolerance to fats (gallbladder problems). Severe anemia. Varicose veins. Has SEX to please partner. Pains caused chilliness. NWS (Never will since) puberty. CHANGEABLE SYMPTOMS.

Mental/Emotional symptoms—timid, submissive, yielding, PEOPLE PLEASER. Wants CONSOLATION, sympathy, and attention. Fears abandonment, full of cares, tells you everything. Indecisive. Laughs or CRIES EASILY. Fears being in a crowd, being alone, being in the dark, and insanity. Indecisive. Demanding. Claustrophobic.

MODALITIES
Worse—warmth, rich foods, FATS, puberty, pregnancy, before menstruation, violent emotions, good cry, hard pressure. Better—COLD, fresh air, standing erect. Time—worse evening.

ASSOCIATED
Sides—RIGHT.
Organs—hypothalamus—hypophysis, thyroid, genitals, adrenals, circulation.
Gender—feminine.
Personalities—secretaries, nurses, housewives, thieves.
Causation—abandonment, eating fats.
Common Health Issues—amenorrhea (lack of menstruation), anemia, chicken pox, conjunctivitis, earaches, ear problems, eye problems, gallbladder problems, leucorrhea (vaginal discharge), measles, mumps, loss of smell, vaginitis.

PYROGENIUM
Pyrogenium (Rotten meat pus)

KEYNOTES
INFECTIONS, BAD SMELLING DISCHARGES, FEVERS with sepsis.

SYMPTOMS
Physical symptoms—offensive smell of saliva and mucus discharges. All DISCHARGES BAD-SMELLING. Fevers, chills. Fever with sore limbs. HIGH FEVER above 103 degrees. PULSE TOO QUICK—heart palpitations. Blood poisoning. Sepsis infection. Bed sores. BRUISED SENSATION. Menstruation has offensive smell. Exhausted and Restless. Wants a hot bath. All symptoms worse cold.

Mental/Emotional symptoms—talkative, especially during fever. Feels the heart consciously. Confused identity. Bed feels too hard. Desires to be rocked. Restless. Delirium. Anxious.

MODALITIES
Worse—cold damp, passing gas, night. Better—hot bath, heat, pressure. Time—worse night.

ASSOCIATED
Sides—either.

Organs—blood, heart, circulation, muscles.

Gender—masculine or feminine.

Personalities—not important.

Causation—infection with pus, miscarriage, chronic diseases.

Common Health Issues—abscesses, bed sores, bites: insect or animal, blood poisoning, fevers, heart palpitations, infections, lymphatic in-flammation, offensive discharges, wounds.

RANUNCULUS
Ranunculus Bulbosus (Buttercup)

KEYNOTES
RIB NERVE INJURY, SHINGLES, LEFT SHOULDER.

SYMPTOMS
Physical symptoms—bluish herpes on face. COLD SORES. Allergies—hay fever. LEFT SCAPULA PAIN. Cold chest and sternum. Bruised sternum. Nerve pains between the ribs from lung problems mainly left-sided, or from injury, bruising or breaking. Intercostal rib neuralgia (nerve pain) after shingles. SHINGLES with bluish skin itching or itching from contact. CHILLY BODY. Stitching and shooting pains. Bruised soreness. Alcoholism. Pains are worse by pressure.

Mental/Emotional symptoms—scolding, irritable, hasty. Delirium tremens. Mental effects of alcoholism.

MODALITIES
Worse—AIR, changes, alcohol, evening, breathing, touch, wet stormy weather, after eating. Better—belching, rest, warmth, warm weather. Time—worse mornings.

ASSOCIATED
Sides—right.

Organs—skin, muscles, ribs, lungs, nerves.

Gender—masculine or feminine.

Personalities—seamstresses, secretaries, computer work, piano players.

Causation—rib injury.

Common Health Issues—alcoholism, delirium tremens, hangover, shingles, rib pains, neuralgia nerve pain.

RHUS TOX
Rhus Tox (Poison Oak)

KEYNOTES
STIFFNESS BETTER FROM CONTINUED MOTION, CRACKING
JOINTS, WORSE BEFORE STORMS.

SYMPTOMS
Physical symptoms—bags under eyes. Cold sores (herpes zoster).
Obesity. Cracking vertebrae. Spinal injuries. Joint injuries, dislocations,
tendonitis. Greasy skin. Picks at clothes. Plays with fingers. Rashes. Stiff
and restless, hard to sleep. Stretching.
Mental/Emotional symptoms—restlessness. Anxiety at night. Timid.

MODALITIES
Worse—cold, damp, wet, rainy, before storms, drafts, beginning motion, rest, injuries, NIGHT. Better—continued motion, heat, stretching,
rubbing. Time—worse night.

ASSOCIATED
Sides—left.
Organs—muscles, tendons, ligaments, joints, spine, skin.
Gender—masculine or feminine.
Personalities—athlete, outside workers.
Causation—spinal or joint injury, cold stormy weather, getting wet.
Common Health Issues—arthritis, injuries, rashes, spinal injuries—es-
pecially lower back.

RUMEX
Rumex Crispus (Yellow dock)

KEYNOTES
DRY SPASMODIC COUGH, everything is worse from EXPOSURE TO COLD AIR.

SYMPTOMS
Physical symptoms—acts like Ferrum phos (iron). Cheeks flushed red. Allergies—hay fever. Loss of voice when cold. Tickling in pit of throat. Lymphatics enlarged. Chilly. Rashes. Lungs raw or burning. Cough tickling in throat. Dry spasmodic COUGH, winter, daytime, 11 P.M. or 2 A.M. Cold hands when coughing. Dry, hacking, tickling cough. Cough worse from slightest cold air or uncovering. Excessive discharges. Diarrhea in morning. Everything worse from CHANGE OF TEMPERATURE and COLD AIR.

Mental/Emotional symptoms—sad. Serious. Apathetic. Fears misfortune.

MODALITIES
Worse—inhaling COOL AIR, pressure, uncovering or undressing, lying on left side. Better—wrapping head, warmth, covering mouth. Time—11 P.M. or 2 A.M. dry cough.

ASSOCIATED
Sides—either.

Organs—respiratory, intestines, nerves, joints, ankles.

Gender—masculine or feminine.

Personalities—not important.

Causation—lung weakness, exposure to COLD AIR.

Common Health Issues—anemia, bronchitis, coughs, gas, throat disorders.

RUTA

Ruta Graveolens (Garden rue)

KEYNOTES

TENDONITIS, INJURY, WORSE FROM TOUCH.

SYMPTOMS

Physical symptoms—eye, retinal detachment. Divergent strabismus (eyeballs go to opposite sides). Unquenchable thirst. Vertebrae slips out. Deforming arthritis of hands. Wrist as if strained. Sprains of wrists and ankles. Carpal tunnel. Ganglion cyst. INJURIES. Nodules after injury. Bursitis. Tendonitis. Lameness after strains. Inflammation of periosteum (bone membrane covering). #1 remedy for trigger finger or finger dupuytren contracture (Causticum). Sciatica. Legs give out on rising. Prolapsed rectum. Aversion to motion.

Mental/Emotional symptoms—self-dissatisfaction, feeling defeated, doubts success. Nervous at the slightest touch. Wants to contradict. Weakness. Despair. Intense apathy.

MODALITIES

Worse—strain (especially eyestrain), cold, damp, lying, sitting, stooping, straining at stool. Better—lying on back, warmth, daytime. Time—worse on waking, better in daytime.

ASSOCIATED

Sides—right.

Organs—periosteum, eyes fibrous, connective tissue, eye muscles, tendons, ligaments.

Gender—masculine or feminine.

Personalities—construction workers, athletes.

Causation—injuries, tendon overuse, hamstrings.

Common Health Issues—arthritis, backache, bone bruises, carpal tunnel, eyestrain, ganglion cysts, joints dislocate, lameness, sprains, tendonitis.

SABADILLA
Sabadilla Officinalis (Cevadilla seed)

KEYNOTES
Allergies/hay fever, sneezing—worse smells, cold air, PARASITES, MUCUS—thin.

SYMPTOMS
Physical symptoms—eyes, tears. ALLERGIES/HAYFEVER, SNEEZING —very sensitive to smells. SPASMODIC REPETITIVE SNEEZING with mucus, running nose, tears in eyes. Lots of clear mucus, nose itches. Sweet taste in mouth. Craves hot things. No thirst. Can't stick out tongue with sore throat. Constant desire to swallow. Cough on first lying down. Parasites—pinworms. Thickened toenails change sides. Feels chilly, sensitive to cold air.

Mental/Emotional symptoms—strange imaginations, confused identity. Large sense of guilt. Hard to focus. Worse thinking of complaints. Laughs or is apathetic, thinking causes sleeplessness and headaches.

MODALITIES
Worse—cold, time periods, before midnight, resting, odors. Better— open air, wrapping up, warmth, swallowing, eating. Time—worse before midnight, and periodically.

ASSOCIATED
Sides—right to left.

Organs—mucus membrane, tear ducts, nose, anus.

Gender—masculine or feminine.

Personalities—not important.

Causation—mental overwork, parasites causing convulsions, nymphomania (hypersexuality).

Common Health Issues—allergies—hay fever, chilliness, mucus, lice, pinworms, parasites, sneezing.

SABAL
Sabal Serrulata (Saw palmetto)

KEYNOTES
BREASTS, PROSTATE, SEXUAL problems.

SYMPTOMS
Physical symptoms—hirsutism (dark, coarse, facial hair in women). Craves milk. Woman-breasts small and atrophied (from breastfeeding), underdeveloped, or atrophy of one breast. Obesity. Pains are sharp and stinging. Back ache after sex. Male-prostate enlargement (BPH) with urging, dribbling at night; sperm at stool or urination; painful sex, desire diminished. Cold or heat in genitals.

Mental/Emotional symptoms—apathy. Aversion to company. Thinks only of their own problems. Fears of falling asleep. Doesn't want to be consoled. Loss of sexual desire.

MODALITIES
Worse—cold, damp, cloudy, waking, sympathy, before menstruation. Better—sleep, milk. Time—worse early morning, or late afternoon to night.

ASSOCIATED
Sides—either.

Organs—genital, urinary, breasts, mucus membranes.

Gender—masculine or feminine.

Personalities—not important.

Causation—sexual excesses.

Common Health Issues—bedwetting, BPH (enlarged prostate), epididymitis (male genital inflammation), hirsutism (excess facial hair in women), prostatitis, sexual debility, urinary incontinence, urinary tract infection (UTI).

SANGUINARIA
Sanguinaria Canadensis (Blood root)

KEYNOTES
RIGHT-SIDED EVERYTHING, ESPECIALLY HEADACHES, MUCUS BURNING SENSATIONS.

SYMPTOMS
Physical symptoms—arthritis. Headache right side. Migraine, right side, with vomiting every seventh day—starts shoulder, neck to right temple to right eye—comes and goes with the sun, better in a quiet dark room, also with veins of temples distended. Allergies—hay fever. Sick from smell of flowers. Nasal polyps. Mucus. Nausea on blowing nose. Acrid or irritating discharges. Red face. Red cheeks. Cheeks burning. Right deltoid rheumatism. Whooping cough after flu in children. Menopausal symptoms—headaches, hot flashes, vaginal discharges. Burning sensations. Burning palms or soles of feet. Warm blooded.

Mental/Emotional symptoms—anxious, paralyzed emotionally, sensitive to noise.

MODALITIES
Worse—periodically, menopause, light, raising arms, sweating, odors, jarring, motion. Better—sleeping, vomiting, cool air, urination, passing gas, belching, sitting up, dark room. Time—worse with the sun, and at night.

ASSOCIATED
Sides—right.

Organs—lung (right), chest, liver, nose, eustachian tube (right).

Gender—masculine or feminine.

Personalities—not important.

Causation—after whooping cough, taking cold from sweating.

Common Health Issues—blood disorders, headaches, gallbladder, polyps, arthritis-especially right shoulder, sinusitis.

SECALE
Secale Cornutum (Orgot of rye)

KEYNOTES
HEMORRHAGES, PASSIVE BLEEDING (slow bleeding), WORSE HEAT.

SYMPTOMS
Physical symptoms—large appetite, wants cold drinks or ice. Burning discharges. HOT, burning, but skin feels cold. Violent and crampy pains. Ice cold. Progression of skin boils to pus, then greenish pustules, then gangrene. Skin feels like crawling ants. Arteriosclerosis. Raynaud's disease (lack of circulation in hands). Hemorrhages (excess bleeding), oozing watery blood. Threatened miscarriage. Female: brownish offensive vaginal discharges. Sensitive to noise. Numbness. All symptoms are worse in warm air. Insomnia from abuse of drugs.

Mental/Emotional symptoms—restless, sarcastic, confused. Shameless, mocking. Irritable. Suspicious. Forgetful after sex.

MODALITIES
Worse—menstruation, pregnancy, fluid loss, after eating, covering, heat, miscarriage. Better—doubled up, cold, rocking, stretching, rubbing, after vomiting. Time—not important.

ASSOCIATED
Sides—RIGHT.

Organs—uterus, blood, nerves, muscles.

Gender—feminine, women who are flabby or emaciated.

Personalities—alcohol or drug abuse.

Causation—miscarriage, hemorrhages (excess bleeding), suppression of discharges.

Common Health Issues—gangrene, hemorrhages (excess bleeding), locomotor Ataxia (can't walk properly), miscarriage, nosebleeds, Raynaud's disease (cold hands), vaginal discharge.

SELENIUM
Selenium (element Selenium)

KEYNOTES
IMPOTENCE, sensitive to drafts.

SYMPTOMS
Physical symptoms—hair loss, everywhere. Pain in the hair when touched. Voice hoarse. Craving alcohol. Liver enlarged, rash on skin above liver. Oily skin. Psoriasis in palms of hands. Weakness after acute or recent disease. Drunk easily. Male: increased sexual desire brings impotence; prostatitis, weakness from hard stool; sperm loss without ejaculation. Itching ankles. Sensitive to drafts. Emaciation. Weakness after fever or alcohol.

Mental/Emotional symptoms—theorizes, fanatical, mind exhaustion, fatigue. Religious contemplation. Extreme sadness, depression. Worse thinking about sex, feels conflicted.

MODALITIES
Worse—singing, draft, after sleep, sun, summer, wine, mental effort and physical exertion, alcohol, touch. Better—cold air, drinking cold water, rest, after sunset. Time—better afternoons, after sunset.

ASSOCIATED
Sides—LEFT.
Organs—nerves, larynx, genitals, urinary.
Gender—masculine.
Personalities—singers, teachers with voice issues.
Causation—sexual excess, debilitating events, drug use or abuse, over study.
Common Health Issues—hair loss, impotence, prostate problems, low sperm count.

Sepia

SEPIA
Sepia Succus (Cuttlefish Ink)

KEYNOTES
Athletic, tall, dark hair, craves sour foods, low sex drive, family is DUTY only, HORMONAL PROBLEMS.

SYMPTOMS
Physical symptoms—greasy skin, rings under eyes, Cholasma (brown spots) or yellow saddle over nose. Teen acne. Facial warts, dark hair. Hirsutism (excess facial hair in women) (Ignatia, Sabal, Thuja). Lump in throat (Ignatia). Craves sour foods and chocolate. Morning sickness. Alcohol or sexual excesses. Sore liver. Talks with hands. When warn out they become fat, angry, with no sex drive. Aversion to breastfeeding—it is draining for them. Big family. Must exercise to feel better. Menstruation scanty flow. Worse from hysterectomy. Hair falls out at menopause. Fallen uterus. Weak lower back. Genital warts. Sensation as if ball in rectum. Tall, thin person with narrow pelvis, flat chested. Masculine walk, moves shoulders instead of hips. Thick greenish discharges. Oversensitive to noise.

Mental/Emotional symptoms—dancers, love to dance. Low sex drive, wants to be alone, does family duties, inability to give love and affection. Aversion to sex, worse from consolation. Cries from telling her symptoms, confusion. Indifference to loved ones. Inability to love or give affection. Aversion to sex, no orgasms, fears rape and men, history of sexual abuse. Hates consolation. Better when busy, wants to be independent. Spiteful before menstruation. Hormonal disturbances. Intuitive, but introverted (Phosphorus=extrovert). In later stages is fat, critical and emotionally cold.

MODALITIES
Worse—cold, before menstruation, pregnancy, eating, afternoon, 5 P.M., milk, menopause. Better—dancing, warmth, motion, cold drinks,

crossing legs, loosening clothes, open air. Times—worse 5 P.M., after-noon, better evenings.

ASSOCIATED

Sides—left.

Organs—female genital circulation, digestive, adrenals, genitals, uterus, nerves, skin.

Gender—feminine, mostly female (10 percent male).

Personalities—women athletes, spiritual leaders, workaholics, managers, dancers.

Causation—hormonal imbalances (estrogen), birth control medications, pregnancy, childbirth, sexual abuse, abortion, or anything else that causes changes to hormones.

Common Health Issues—hormonal disorders, morning sickness, infertility, menopause disorders, uterine prolapse, vaginitis, female cancers, Addison's disease (adrenals), baby fat (Calc carb), constipation during pregnancy (calc carb, alum).

SILICEA
Silicea (Silicon Dioxide)

KEYNOTES
Shy, perfectionist, scars easily, poor fingernails, every injury goes to pus, infections.

SYMPTOMS
Physical symptoms—large head. Thin hair. Excess earwax. Earaches. Teeth problems, weak. Hair on tongue sensation. Hates warm foods and milk. Sour-smelling sweat. Swollen abdomen. Thin fingernails. Thin limbs. Skin-thin pus, scars easily. Hard lumps. Constipation at menstruation. Delicate, thin, frail, pale person. Weakness from vaccinations.

Mental/Emotional symptoms—students, mental overwork. Procrastinator, lack of follow-through or stamina. Perfectionist. Timid, bashful. Fears of needles or sharp objects.

MODALITIES
Worse—cold, drafts, light, noise, night, menstruation, vaccinations, milk. Better—warmth, urination. Time—not important.

ASSOCIATED
Sides—either.

Organs—nerves, bones, skin, mucus membranes.

Gender—masculine or feminine.

Personalities—artists, healers, mathematicians, office workers, over-workers, homeopaths, lawyers, students.

Causation—vaccinations, injuries, foreign objects in the body (splinters, etc.).

Common Health Issues—pus formation, scoliosis—crooked spine (Calc fluor), skin problems, splinter removal, scars.

SPIGELIA
Spigelia Anthelmintica (Pinkroot)

KEYNOTES
MIGRAINES LEFT-SIDE, TOBACCO AGGRAVATES, VIOLENT PAINS.

SYMPTOMS
Physical symptoms—migraine—left eye beneath eyebrow and temple, better with cold applications, or feels like a band around the head. GLAUCOMA in the left eye. TRIGEMINAL NEURALGIA (facial nerve pain) left side. Heart palpitations can be heard through the chest, often occurring with eye symptoms. HEART SYMPTOMS—angina, craving hot water. Violent pains. Bad breath. GOITER. Tobacco aggravates. Fingernails are brittle (Silicea). MENSTRUATION too early. Chilly body, worse cold.

Mental/Emotional symptoms—fear of pointy objects, stuttering, responsible people. Restless. Nervous agitation. Anxiety. Can't tolerate thinking of pain. Delusions of seeing PINS or sharp objects.

MODALITIES
Worse—touch, motion, tobacco, sex, noise, turning eyes, stooping, stormy weather. Better—cold applications (headache), dry weather, rest. Time—worse with sun, better after sunset.

ASSOCIATE
Sides—left.

Organs—nerves, eyes, teeth.

Gender—masculine or feminine.

Personalities—not important.

Causation—head injury, parasites, sun exposure, tobacco.

Common Health Issues—angina (heart pain), anxiety, eye pains, eye problems, heart disorders, heart palpitations, migraines, trigeminal neuralgia (face pain).

SPONGIA
Spongia tosta (Roasted sponge)

KEYNOTES
THYROID, HEART, WORSE COLD and DRY, SUFFOCATION SENSATION.

SYMPTOMS
Physical symptoms—throat, as if plug in larynx. Thirsty. Hungry. Thyroid disease. Goiter. Croupy cough with anxiety from difficult breathing. Asthma—dryness, suffocation, worse in dry cold. Heart palpitations, angina (heart pain), heart-valve disease, may also help in heart failure. Indigestion from pancreas problems. Pancreatitis. Skin dryness. Chronic testicular pain. Chilly body. Better warm foods, drinks.

Mental/Emotional symptoms—fears of heart disease and suffocation. Averse to change. Talkative. Moody. Loves to sing. Anxiety with difficult breathing.

MODALITIES
Worse—cold, dry, wind, waking up, physical exertion, touch, thinking of symptoms, pressure, atmospheric pressure. Better—descending (going down stairs), bending forward, drinking, rest. Time—worse midnight, 12-2 A.M., and after sleep.

ASSOCIATED
Sides—left.

Organs—heart, larynx, throat, thyroid, pancreas, testicles, nerves, lymph.

Gender—masculine or feminine.

Personalities—not important.

Causation—fibroid problems.

Common Health Issues—croupy cough, physical exhaustion, goiter, heart failure, indigestion (pancreas), thyroid disorders, whooping cough.

STANNUM MET
Stannum Metallicum (Tin)

KEYNOTES
LUNG WEAKNESS, WEAKNESS, WEAK VOICE.

SYMPTOMS
Physical symptoms—bitter taste. Smell of cooking causes nausea and vomiting. Any lung problem (asthma, pneumonia, etc.) with weak feeling, can hardly talk. Exhausting night sweats. Stomach feels empty. Emaciation. Pains gradually increase or decrease. Paralysis, heaviness, weakness. Limbs give way when trying to sit down. Trembling from weakness.

Mental/Emotional symptoms—anxiousness, sadness, discouraged. Moody. Feels worse when weeping. Lung problems cause depression. Fears of people, society, crowds. Sadness before menstruation. Wants to be alone.

MODALITIES
Worse—using voice, laughing, talking, going downstairs, from stool. Better—walking, pressure, bending double, rapid motion. Time— worse at 10 A.M.

ASSOCIATED
Sides—left.

Organs—lungs, mucus membranes, nerves.

Gender—masculine or feminine.

Personalities—not important.

Causation—voice overuse, teething, emotions, masturbation.

Common Health Issues—bronchitis, hoarseness, lung weakness, weak voice, vertigo going downstairs.

STAPHYSAGRIA
Delphinium Staphysagria (Stavesacre)

KEYNOTES
HISTORY OF SEXUAL ABUSE, CHRONIC UTIs from SEX, SURGICAL CUTS, ROTTEN EGG SMELL.

SYMPTOMS
Physical symptoms—styes around eyes leave hard nodules. Gums bleed easily. Tooth decay—dark, decayed edges, sensitive to dental procedures. Insect stings, lice. Honeymoon cystitis—from sex. Can't have sex without antibiotics because of UTI (urinary tract infection). Surgical wounds. Odors of rotten eggs (Sulphur). Surgical cuts.

Mental/Emotional symptoms—overly sweet, nice, considerate, sensitive, vulnerable. Appears masculine, hard. Victim. Avoids confrontation, yielding resignation, don't fight for their rights. Worried about injustice. Hates authority. Want to please you. Blushes easily. Disappointed love, romantic disappointment. Emotionally stuck, frustration. ANGER, throws things. Personal pride and keeping a sense of honor. History of rape, battered wife, sexually abused child. Guilt, shame. Fear of intimacy with masturbation, or sexually promiscuous. Fears of losing control. Addiction to drugs.

MODALITIES
Worse—emotions from remembering abuse or humiliation, sexual excess, masturbation, cold drinks, wounds, night, mornings, tobacco. Better—breakfast, warmth, rest. Time—worse mornings.

ASSOCIATED
Sides—RIGHT.
Organs—genitals, urinary, teeth, nervous system, liver.
Gender—more feminine, victims.
Personalities—introverted artists, priests.
Causation—shame, punishment, humiliation, rape, surgery.
Common Health Issues—anger-suppressed, colic, colitis, eyelid problems, humiliation, masturbation, rape, sexual excess, styes, surgery, UTI (urinary tract infection).

STRAMONIUM
Datura Stramonium* (Jimsom weed)

KEYNOTES
Night terrors, victims of violence, PTSD.

SYMPTOMS
Physical symptoms—seizures. Throat feels closed in. Loss of voice after anger. Teeth turn black. Coughs from tobacco smoke. Slow injury-repair, never well since surgery. Urinary tract infections, especially after intercourse (Staphysagria). Hemophilia (bleeds easily). Hypoglycemia (low blood sugar).

Mental/Emotional symptoms—overly sweet, nice, considerate. Avoids confrontation, yielding, resignation, people-pleaser. Masculine, but soft and sensitive. No bitterness. Blushes easily. Incoherent speech, stuttering. Overtalkative. Doesn't express feelings openly. Violence or victim of violence. Fears of dark and imminent danger. Nightmares (terrors), PTSD (post traumatic stress disorder). Religious obsessions.

MODALITIES
Worse—shiny objects, from sleep, darkness, cloudy days, being alone, swallowing liquids, being touched. Better—light, warmth, cold water, company of others. Time—worse during sleep (nightmares).

ASSOCIATED
Sides—either.

Organs—genito-urinary organs, teeth, nervous system, liver, mind, muscles.

Gender—masculine or feminine. Personalities—introverted painters, musicians, priest. Causation—exposure to violence, getting wet, electricity.

Common Health Issues—nightmares, nosebleeds, pneumonia, PTSD (post-traumatic stress disorder), victims of violence.

*Not in found in Conditions chapter.

SULPHUR
Sulphur (element Sulphur)

KEYNOTES
Rotten-egg smell, extrovert, intellectual.

SYMPTOMS
Physical symptoms—arrogant look on face. Sweaty smell. Asthma alternating with eczema. Talks in monologue. #1 remedy for digestive ulcers. Wringing hands. Rotten-egg gas. #1 remedy for pneumonia. Untidy and unwashed person. Odd clothing choices. Physically awkward. Odd gestures. Sleep—laughs, walks, talks.

Mental/Emotional symptoms—dreamers, philosophers, inventors, rush of too many ideas—can't accomplish anything. Vain, self-centered. Argumentative, collects things, hoarder, or trash looks beautiful to them. Fear of heights.

MODALITIES
Worse bathing, heat, weather changes, 11 A.M., early morning, full moon, speaking. Better—open air, warm drinks, sweating, lying on right side. Time—worse 11 A.M.

ASSOCIATED
Sides—left.

Organs—SKIN, endocrine glands.

Gender—More masculine.

Personalities—business persons, engineers, inventors, professors, charlatans, homeopaths. Causation—alcoholism, never will since taking purgatives, never will since pneumonia.

Common Health Issues—eczema, digestive ulcers, gas, pneumonia.

SULPHURIC ACID
Sulphuricum Acidum (Vitriol)

KEYNOTES
INJURIES, especially eyes and brain, HEAT, MENOPAUSE SYMPTOMS.

SYMPTOMS
Physical symptoms—right temples. ABSORBS BLEEDING, especially in eyes and brain. Larynx moves up and down violently. Sourness, belching, heartburn. Weakness from excess sweating. Bruising easily. Gangrene. Trembling internally, tremors. Menopause symptoms including hot flashes. Injuries with bleeding. Hot flashes with sweating. Chilly body, worst cold. Worse from smoke in air or smoking. Pains come and go suddenly.

Mental/Emotional symptoms—always in a hurry, can't calm down. Must be on time. Not patient with others. Confused while sitting. Alcoholism—cravings.

MODALITIES
Worse—coffee smell, menopause, open-air, sleep, too much heat, cold. Better—hands over head, hot drinks, lying on affected side. Time—worse evening, late morning, sleep.

ASSOCIATED
Sides—RIGHT.

Organs—blood, digestive tract.

Gender—masculine or feminine.

Personalities—not important.

Causation—burns, injuries, surgical operations.

Common Health Issues—alcoholism, brain or eye bleeding, bruises, burns, gangrene, heartburn, hot flashes, ulcers.

SYMPHYTUM
Symphytum Officinale (Comfrey)

KEYNOTES
BONE INJURIES, BLUNT TRAUMA INJURIES.

SYMPTOMS
Physical symptoms—eyeball trauma. Bone fractures—accelerates
bone growth. Prickling pain at bone fracture. Painful old bone injuries. Injuries from blunt force. Bone fractures, non-union (not healing),
compound. Periosteum injuries. Tendonitis. Phantom limb pains. First
aid for bone fractures.
Mental/Emotional symptoms—dwells on past disagreeable events.

MODALITIES
Worse—injuries, blunt-force, touch, motion, pressure, walking. Better—
warmth, gentle motion. Time—not important.

ASSOCIATED
Sides—either.
Organs—bones, cartilage, periosteum (bone covering).
Gender—masculine or feminine.
Personalities—not important.
Causation—broken bones, injuries, blunt trauma injuries (being hit by
something hard).
Common Health Issues—bone fractures, bone injuries, eye injuries,
gunshot wounds, phantom limb pain.

TABACUM
Nicotiana tabacum (Tobacco)

KEYNOTES
MOTION SICKNESS, NAUSEA, VERTIGO.

SYMPTOMS
Physical symptoms—VISION problems with temporary vision loss. MOTION SICKNESS with nausea and vomiting in spasms with sinking feeling. Morning sickness. Cold sweat worse with smell of tobacco. Pains come on suddenly. Angina (heart pain). Muscle paralysis. VERTIGO with NAUSEA, sweating, opening eyes. Nausea with spitting, deathly sick.

Mental/Emotional symptoms—acute anxiety. Excitement. Cheerful. Lazy. Anxiety when alone. Feels unfortunate. Depression. Cold sweats worse from tobacco smell.

MODALITIES
Worse—motion, opening eyes, walking, heat. Better—cold air, uncovering abdomen, cold applications, vinegar, vomiting. Time—worse evenings.

ASSOCIATED
Sides—left.

Organs—nerves, heart, glands. Gender—masculine or feminine. Personalities—not important. Causation—Sun exposure, insect bites.

Common Health Issues—fainting, morning sickness, motion sickness, nausea, vertigo, vomiting.

TELLURIUM MET
Tellurium Metallicum (element Tellurium)

KEYNOTES
LOWER SPINE INJURY, RINGWORM, offensive smells and discharges.

SYMPTOMS
Physical symptoms—dry mouth, garlic odor. Wants cold drinks, beer. RINGWORM, especially on the face. Chilly body. Discharges irritating, bad smelling. Offensive body odors. Herniated discs. Contraction of tendons of knees. Sciatica right. Weakness in lumbar vertebrae. Offensive foot sweat.

Mental/Emotional symptoms—fof being touched. Forgetful. Apathetic. Depressed.

MODALITIES
Worse—spinal injuries, cold weather, weekly, swallowing, touch, lying on parts. Better—lying on back in case of back problems. Time—not important.

ASSOCIATED
Sides—left.

Organs—spine, ears, eyes, nerve, skin.

Gender—masculine or feminine.

Personalities—not important.

Causation—INJURIES.

Common Health Issues—coughs, herniated discs, injuries, offensive sweat, ringworm, sacroiliac pain, skin eczema (beard), spinal irritation.

TEREBINTHIA
Terebinthia Oleum (Turpentine)

KEYNOTES
Kidney, urine smells like violets, PAIN causes urination.

SYMPOTMS
Physical symptoms—burning. Bleeding mucus membrane surfaces. Hemorrhages (excess bleeding). Chilly body. Edema (swelling). Bruising. Pain causes urination. Urination has ODOR OF VIOLETS. Nephritis—kidney inflammation. UTIs (urinary tract infections).

Mental/Emotional symptoms—dullness and confusion, better with urination. Anxiety going to bed.

MODALITIES
Worse—damp, cold, lying down, pressure, walking, urination, sitting. Better—motion, walking, belching, turning right, passing gas, stooping. Time—worse night, and worse from 1-3 A.M.

ASSOCIATED
Sides—either.

Organs—KIDNEYS, bladder, LUNGS, heart, blood.

Gender—masculine or feminine.

Personalities—not important.

Causation—alcohol, injuries, tooth extraction, damp cellars.

Common Health Issues—irritable bladder, hemorrhage, kidney problems, nephritis (kidney inflammation), urinary tract infection (UTI), urine retention, painful urination.

THUJA
Thuja Occidentalis (Arbor vitae)

KEYNOTES
Feeling "disgusting," warts, abnormal non-cancerous growths, yellow-greenish discharges.

SYMPTOMS
Physical symptoms—dark-haired. All discharges yellow to green. Unhealthy skin. Greasy or waxy skin. Deep nasolabial lines (extend from either side of nose down to the corners of the mouth). Acne on chin with scarring. Hirsutism—dark, thick, coarse hair on face in women, sometimes chest (Ignatia, Sabal, Sepia). Craves onions or has an aversion to them. Sweat that is sickly-SWEET smelling. Tendency to obesity. #1 remedy for WARTS. Anemic. Non-cancerous growth, especially genital area. #1 remedy for left ovarian cysts (Lachesis, Sepia). Sleep—moan, shriek, sweat, or masturbate. All symptoms worse from fat. Bathes or washes often. Children act like "know it all." Bad effects from vaccinations.

Mental/Emotional symptoms—serious, closed, unemotional, rigid. Misleading. Gives long story without clarity. Obsessive, religious fanaticism. Duty. Polite. Manipulative, Guilt. Secrets about sex, drugs, stealing. Evasive, feels trapped and hides. Low self-esteem, feels ugly. Feels disgusting, like hiding something. Can't find the right words. Dreams of death.

MODALITIES
Worse—cold damp, sun, bright light, night, closing eyes, urinating, sex, vaccinations. Better—motion, drawing or crossing legs, pressure, rubbing, scratching, warmth. Time—worse 3 A.M. or 3 P.M.

ASSOCIATED
Sides—left.
Organs—genitals, urinary, skin.

Gender—masculine or feminine.

Personalities—politicians.

Causation—gonorrhea in the past, arthritis, allergies, never well since vaccinations, spinal injury, from abusive family.

Common Health Issues—cysts, polyps, non-cancerous growths, skin warts, venereal warts, other warts, vaccination effects.

URTICA
Urtica urens (Stinging Nettle)

KEYNOTES
HIVES, RASHES, stinging, burning, SHELLFISH allergy.

SYMPTOMS
Physical symptoms—shellfish allergy. GOUT and arthritis. Right deltoid muscle. Swollen breasts, milk absent. Allergic swelling (edema). First-degree burns, from hot water, with itching. Sunburn. Stings, bites. Hives, intolerable itching with arthritis. Stinging, burning pains. Kidney stones. Chicken pox.

Mental/Emotional symptoms—not important.

MODALITIES
Worse—burns, cool, stings, shellfish, night, arthritis. Better—lying down, rubbing. Time—not important.

ASSOCIATED
Sides—either.

Organs—breasts, genitals, urinary.

Gender—masculine or feminine.

Personalities—not important.

Causation—burn effects, stings, rashes, shellfish.

Common Health Issuses—allergic reactions (especially to shellfish), arthritis, burns, gout, hives, kidney stones, neuritis, rashes.

VERATRUM
Vertram Album (White hellebore)

KEYNOTES
EXCESSIVE DISCHARGES, COLD SWEAT, EMOTIONAL EXTREMES, RELIGIOUS.

SYMPTOMS
Physical symptoms—vertigo with cold sweat. Fainting suddenly. COLD breath. Cold sweating especially in forehead and abdomen. Lean, energetic person. Foolish gestures. Muscle SPASMS and CRAMPS. POST-OPERATIVE shock with cold sweat and low pulse. CHOLERA, or diarrhea with vomiting. Stool, large amounts, and green. All symptoms WORSE SPRING and AUTUMN.

Mental/Emotional symptoms—BOASTING and LYING. Extravagant, AMBITIOUS, flattering. No tact. Irritable. Mania leads to violence or kissing. Obscene or religious. Cheats, pretends. Rude. Injured pride or honor. Dignified. Fears loss of social position.

MODALITIES
Worse—physical exertion, fright, cold wet, menstruation, change of weather, during pain, motion. Better—hot drinks, lying, warm food, stimulants. Time—not important.

ASSOCIATED
Sides—LEFT.

Organs—nerves, GI tract, heart, respiratory.

Gender—masculine or feminine.

Personalities—workaholics, business people, teachers, foreman, gurus, priests.

Causation—post-operative shock, injury, disappointed love or honor, drug abuse.

Common Health Issues—cholera, collapse, coma, dehydration, fainting, head injury, mania, meningitis, shock, sunstroke.

ZINCUM
Zincumum Metallicum (element Zinc)

KEYNOTES
NERVE EXHAUSTION, SPASMS, EMOTIONAL EXHAUSTION.

SYMPTOMS
Physical symptoms—rolls head from side to side. Vertigo. Pale face. Seizures or convulsions with pale face. ALCOHOLISM. Emaciated. MULTIPLE SCLEROSIS. NERVE DISEASES. Burning pains. Pain below the navel. Incontinence. Restless legs. Fidgety feet. All physical and mental symptoms worse with loss of sleep.

Mental/Emotional symptoms—secretive, worse being in the light. Religious. Suppressed emotions. Quiet. Sensitive to noises. Mental exhaustion. COMPLAINERS, moody. Forgetful. Irritable in the evening.

MODALITIES
Worse—physical exhaustion, noise, touch, heat, wine. Better—menstruation, urination, motion, hard pressure, warm open air. Time—worse 11-12 A.M. with hunger, and evening with irritability.

ASSOCIATED
Sides—left.

Organs—spine, nervous system, skin.

Gender—masculine or feminine.

Personalities—not important.

Causation—emotional trauma, caretaking, brain injury, sleep loss.

Common Health Issues—alcoholism, foggy brain, convulsions, epilepsy, headaches, head injuries, meningitis, muscle spasms, nerve weakness, paralysis.

CHAPTER 4

Quick Reference Guides

These guides are your sources for quickly finding:

- **Guide #1:** Top Remedies for Conditions (#1 remedies and other top remedies for conditions)
- **Guide #2:** Keynote Symptoms and their Remedies
- **Guide #3:** Common Health Issues and their Remedies
- **Guide #4:** Causations Producing Conditions
- **Guide #5:** Remedies and their Associated Conditions

Quick Reference Guide #1
Top Remedies for Conditions

In Chapter 2, I detailed 78 Conditions (from A to Z—Abscesses to Warts) that can be addressed by homeopathy. There, I listed the Top (#1) Remedies for each Condition, along with additional remedies that might be useful but are not specific to the Condition.

This **Quick Reference Guide #1** gives you immediate access to these Top Remedies. Keep this Guide handy (bookmark this page, or copy it). When you have time to study more, go back to Chapter 2 and get the whole story.

Abscesses/boils—Calc Sulph, also Hepar Sulph, Silicea

Acne in teenage boys with greasy skin—Thuja

Acne, in young women is worse at menstruation—Sepia

After-surgery gas pains—Carbo Veg

Arthritis—Rhus Tox, also Bryonia

Back pain—Rhus Tox, also Tellurium

Bedwetting, when there are no other indications—Equisetum

Bites and stings—Ledum (#2 Apis Mel)

Bites with pain—Arnica

Bloating—Carbo Veg

Blood in the eyes—Sulphuric acid, also Arnica

Bone injuries—Symphytum

Bruising—Arnica (#2 Ledum)

Burns—Cantharis, also Causticum

Cold sores/fever blisters—Nat Mur (#2 Rhus tox)

Colic—Chamomilla

Cough, rattling—Antimonium tart

Cough, whooping—Drosera (#2 Spongia tosta)

Depression Recent or acute—Ignatia

Depression suicidal—Aurum Met, also Nat sulph

Depression, recent—Ignatia

Diarrhea—Podophyllum

Eyes, blood in—Sulphuric acid, also Arnica

Facial hair (hirsutism)—Sepia

First Aid—Arnica, also Rhus tox, Staphysagria

Gas pains, after-surgery—Carbo Veg

Gout—Colchicum

Grief for death of a loved one—Ignatia, also Nat mur

Hair loss—Sepia

Head injury—Nat Sulph, (always start with Arnica)

Hirsutism (dark thick coarse hair on face)—Sepia

Hot flashes, sweaty—Sepia

Incontinence—Causticum

Injury, any, and soft tissue injuries—Arnica

Joint injuries, worse first movement, better continued motion—Rhus Tox

Mononucleosis—Merc Sol or Vivus

Morning sickness—Ipecac, also Nux vomica

Nausea and vomiting—Tabaccum

Nerve pains—Hypericum

Nose bleeds—Phosphorus

Panic attacks—Argentum Nit (#2 Kali ars)

Plantar warts—Antimonium crud (and is #3 remedy for warts)

Pneumonia, left-sided, feeling worse lying on the left side—Phosphorus

Pneumonia, where there is rattling mucus in the upper chest—Antimonium tart

Rattling cough—Antimonium tart

Sinus—Kali bich (#2 Thuja)

Skin issues—Sulphur

Stiffness worse first motion, better continued motion—Rhus Tox

Suicidal depression—Aurum Met

Surgical cuts—Staphysagria

Teething—Chamomilla

Tendon injuries—Ruta Grav

Throbbing pains—Bryonia

Urinary tract infections—Cantharis

Uterine prolapse—Sepia

Vision and retinal issues—Phosphorus

Vomiting and nausea—Tabaccum

Warts—Thuja (#2 Causticum, #3 Antimonium crud)

Whooping cough—Drosera (#2-Spongia tosta)

Quick Reference Guide #2
Keynote Symptoms and Their Remedies

Keynotes are the leading (or most common) symptoms of each remedy. Here, they are in alphabetic order according to the symptom. Additional remedies have been added, where suitable, which may not appear in the keynotes of that remedy.

Abuse, history of sexual abuse—Staphysagria

Acid-balance in the body—Nat phos

Acne, scarring—Kali brom

Allergic reactions—Apis

Allergies—Arsenicum iod, Sabadilla

Alternates sides—Lac caninum

Alternating moods—Lac caninum

Anal deep skin cracks—Nitric acid

Anaphylactic shock—Apis

Anemia—Ferrum met, Ferrum phos

Ankles water retention—Kali carb

Ankles, weak—Calc carb

Anti-anxiety drugs, uses—Kali ars

Anxiety and fear—Kali ars

Anxiety, about health—Agaricus, also Arsenicum

Anxiety, performance—Argentum nit

Asthma, especially from cold humid conditions—Nat sulph

Athletic—Sepia

Ball, sitting on a ball sensation, as if—Chimaphila

Bedwetting—Benzoic acid, Equisetum

Beer, craves—Kali bich

Better continued motion, stiffness—Rhus tox

Better doubling over—Colocynthis

Better heat—Arsenicum, Colocynthis

Better pressure—Colocynthis

Better walking slowly—Ferrum met

Bipolar—Lachesis(especially in women)

Bites or stings—Ledum, also Apis

Bladder—Equisetum

Bleeding—Ferrum phos, Crocus. See also hemorrhages.

Bleeding, passive (flows slowly, seeping)—Hamamelis, Secale

Bloating—Bovista, Carbo veg, China/cinchona

Blood, dark stringy black—Crocus

Blunt trauma injuries—Symphytum, also Arnica

Body acid-balance—Nat phos

Bones—Calc phos, Fluoric acid, Symphytum

Brain injuries—Sulphuric acid, also Natrum sulph

Breasts—Conium, Lac caninum, Sabal

Breasts, mastitis—Phytolacca dec

Bruising—Arnica, Bellis

Burned out, physically or emotionally—Phosphoric acid

Burning—Apis, Allium, Belladonna Urtica, also Phosphorus

Burning sensation—Arsenicum, Capsicum, also Phosphorus

Burning stinging pains—Cantharis

Burns—Calendula, Cantharis, also Causticum

Cancer (breast and prostate)—Conium

Cancer, family history—Carcinosin

Cankers on tongue—Borax, also Arsenicum

Caretaker—Cocculus, also Ignatia

Chest, mucus rattling in—Antimonium tart

Chest, rattling in 4 to 5 A.M.—Nat sulph

Chronic fatigue—Gelsemium, Phosphoric acid

Cold damp conditions—Dulcamara

Cold sweat—Veratrum

Colic—Chamomilla

Colon pain—Colocynthis

Coma—Opium

Constipation, severe—Alumina, Opium

Convulsions—Cicuta, also Cuprum met

Cough, dry spasmodic—Rumex

Cough, spasmodic—Drosera

Cough, whooping—Drosera

Cracking joints—Rhus tox, also Bryonia

Cramps—Cuprum met, Mag phos

Craves beer—Kali bich

Craves meat—Mag carb

Craves salt—Nat mur

Craves sour foods—Sepia

Crying, hysterical—Ignatia

Dark hair—Sepia

Decay—Kreosotum

Dehydration, never well since—China/cinchona

Depression—Aurum met, Cimicifuga, Kali phos, also Ignatia, Nat mur

Diabetes—Lactic acid

Diarrhea—Mercury corrosive, Podophyllum

Digestive disturbances—Mag mur

Discharges, bad smelling—Pyrogenium

Discharges, excessive—Veratrum

Discharges, irritating—Allium

Discharges, white—Kali mur

Discharges, yellow—Nat phos, Nat sulph

Discharges, yellow green—Kali Bich, Mercury sol, Thuja

Disgusting, feeling—Thuja

Dry heaves—Ipecac

Dry or dryness—Alumina, Belladonna, Bryonia, Nat mur

Duty—Kali carb

Ecstasy—Agaricus

Emaciated—Alumina

Emotional exhaustion—Zincum

Emotional extremes—Mercury sol, Veratrum

Emotionally burned out—Phosphoric acid

Enamel(teeth) deficient—Calc fluor

Epilepsy—Calc ars, also Cicuta, Cuprum met

Erotic behavior—Hyoscyamus

Eustachian tube blockage—Kali mur

Excess saliva—Mercury corrosive, Ipecac

Excessive fluids— Lactic acid

Excitement—Agaricus, also Phosphorus

Exhaustion—Carbo veg, Muriatic acid

Exhaustion, emotional—Zincum, also Phosphoric acid

Exhaustion, nerve—Zincum

Exhaustion, physical—Picric acid

Extrovert—Sulphur, also Phosphorus

Eye injuries—Sulphuric acid, also Arnica, Phosphorus

Eye remedy—Euphrasia, also Allium cepa

Eye, central vision disturbance—Carboneum sulph

Eye, excess eye mucus—Euphrasia

Eye, tears bland—Allium

Eye, tears burning—Euphrasia

Eye, vision problems—Cicuta

Family is duty only—Sepia

Fears abandonment—Pulsatilla

Fears about health—Arsenicum

Feeling "disgusting"—Thuja

Female complaints—Lilium tig, also Sepia, Pulsatilla, Lilium tig

Fever—Ferrum phos, Kali sulph, Pyrogenium, also Belladonna

Fingernails, poor—Silicea

Fingers, fidgety—Kali brom

Fluid loss, never will since—China/cinchona

Fluids, lacking—Lactic acid

Fright—Aconite, Gelsemium

Fungal skin problems—Dulcamara

Gas—Carbo veg, China/cinchona, Kali carb, Lycopodium

Glands—Clematis, Phytolacca dec

Gout—Benzoic acid, Colchicum

Grief—Ignatia, Nat mur, Phosphoric acid

Growths, abnormal non-cancerous—Thuja

Hands, wringing—Kali brom

Hard, organs or tissues—Calc fluor

Hay fever—Sabadilla, Arsenicum

Head injury—Cicuta, Helleborus, NAT SULPH, Sulphuric acid

Headaches—Sanguinaria, also Ignatia. See Migraines

Health fears—Arsenicum

Heart—Calc ars, Digitalis, Lilium tig, Spongia

Heartburn—Nat phos

Heat—Sulphuric acid, also Sulphur

Hemorrhoids—Aesculus

Hemorrhages—Crotalus horr, Ferrum met, Hamamelis, Phosphorus, Secale

High blood pressure (hypertension)—Aurum met

Hips—Aesculus

Hives—Urtica

Homesickness—Capsicum

Hormonal—Cimicifuga, Sepia, also Pulsatilla, Lilium tig

Hot—Belladonna, Arsenicum iod

Hydration, water balance—Nat mur

Hysterical rage—Lilium tig

Icy cold person—Carbo veg

Idealist—Causticum

Impotence—Selenium

Infection—Kali bich, Mercury corrosive, Mercury sol, Pyrogenium, Silicea

Inferiority complex—Lycopodium

Inflammation—Ferrum phos

Injuries—Arnica, Bellis, Hypericum perf, Ruta, Sulphuric acid, Symphytum, Tellurium met, also Rhus tox

Injuries, blunt trauma—Symphytum

Injuries, eye—Sulphuric acid

Injury, every one goes to pus—Silicea

Insect bites or stings—Ledum, also Apis

Intellectual—Sulphur

Introvert—Aurum met, Nat mur

Intuitive—China/cinchona, also Phosphorus, Lachesis, Sepia

Irritable—Calc phos, Chamomilla, Nux vomica, also Colocynthis

Joints cracking—Rhus tox, also Bryonia

Keloid scars—Graphites

Kidney—Terebinthina, Berberis vulg

Kidney left—Berberis vulg

Kidney stones—Berberis vulg

Kidneys disease—Calc ars

Lameness—Bellis

Laryngitis—Drosera

Left shoulder—Ranunculus

Life changes—Calc phos

Liver—Digitalis, Lycopodium, Nat sulph, Phosphorus, also Nux Vomica

Lower back—Aesculus, also Tellurium, Hypericum

Lung weakness—Stannum met

Macular degeneration with bleeding—Bovista

Male health, related to emotional/psychological issues—Nux vomica

Mastitis, breasts—Phytolacca dec

Materialistic—Conium, Fluoric acid, also Bryonia

Meat, craves—Mag carb

Menopause—Cimicifuga, Sulphuric acid, also Sepia, Pulsatilla, Graphites

Mental exhaustion—Picric acid, also Phosphoric acid

Metallic smell—Mercury sol

Metallic taste—Mercury sol

Migraines—Glonoinum, Iris versicolor, Spigelia

Milk aggravates or intolerance—Antimonium tart, Mag mur

Mind racing, sleeplessness—Coffea

Mind, overactive—Coffea

Morning sickness—Ipecac, Lactic acid, also Nux vomica

Motion sickness—Cocculus, Petroleum, Tabacum

Mucus—Allium, Arsenicum iod, Kali mur, Sabadilla, Sanguinaria

Mucus rattling in chest—Antimonium tart

Mucus, irritating—Arsenicum iod

Nausea—Antimonium tart, Ipecac, Lactic acid, Lobelia, Tabacum, also Nux vomica

Neck stiffness—Cimicifuga

Nerve exhaustion—Zincum

Nerve injuries—Hypericum perf

Nervous irritability—Kali phos

Nervous system—Kali phos, also Ignatia

Nervousness—Agaricus, also Argentum nit, Gelsemium

Neurological diseases—Cocculus

Night terrors—Stramonium

Noise sensitive—Borax

Obesity—Calc ars, Calc carb, Capsicum, Graphites, Hyoscyamus, Kali carb

Odors, smells of old cheese—Hepar sulph

Offensive discharges—Kreosotum, Tellurium met

Offensive smells—Tellurium met

Old(elderly)—Alumina

Organized overly—Arsenicum, Carcinosin

Organs too hard or too soft—Calc fluor

Overtraining—Arnica

Overwork—Calc carb

Pacifists—Mag mur

Pain from anger—Colocynthis

Pain from frustration—Colocynthis

Pain, bruised—Ledum, also Arnica

Pain, burning—Phosphorus

Pain, causes urination—Terebinthina

Pain, colon—Colocynthis

Pain, intolerable—Chamomilla

Pain, lack of—Opium

Pain, neuralgic—Clematis

Pain, post-shingles—Mezereum

Pain, post-shingles—Mezereum

Pain, radiating—Berberis vulg

Pain, sharp, worse with motion—Bryonia

Pain, shooting—Hypericum perf, Mag phos

Pain, splinter—Hepar sulph, Nitric acid

Pain, violent—Spigelia

Pain, wandering—Berberis vulg, Lac caninum, also Pulsatilla

Pale—Ferrum met

Palpitations on least movement—Digitalis

Pancreas disease—Calc ars

Pancreatitis—Iris versicolor, also Spongia tosta

Panic attacks—Argentum nit, Gelsemium, Kali ars

Paralysis—Causticum

Parasites—Nat phos, Sabadilla

Passionate—Carcinosin

Passive bleeding (flows slowly, seeping)—Hamamelis, Secale

Passive-aggressive—Nux vomica

People pleaser—Pulsatilla

Perfectionist—Silicea

Performance anxiety—Argentum nit

Pessimism—Cimicifuga

Physical exhaustion—Picric acid

Physically, burned out—Phosphoric acid

Post shingles pain—Mezereum

Pregnancy—Cimicifuga

Prolapse—Podophyllum

Prostate—Chimaphila, Conium, Sabal

PTSD (post-traumatic stress disorder)—Stramonium, also Staphysagria

Pulse Slow—Digitalis

Pus—Calc sulph, Mezereum, also Pyrogenium, Silicea

Pus, anywhere there is an abrasion or wound, yellow thick lumpy—Calc sulph

Pus, thick yellow green—Hepar sulph

Rage, hysterical—Lilium tig

Rashes—Urtica

Red—Apis, Belladonna

Religiosity versus sexual excesses—Kali brom

Religious—Veratrum

Restless—Arsenicum iod

Rib nerve injury—Ranunculus

Right-sided—Belladonna, Crotalus horr (like a right-sided Lachesis), Sanguinaria, also Lycopodium

Ringworm—Tellurium met

Rotten egg smell—Staphysagria, Sulphur

Saliva, excess—Mercury corrosive, Ipecac

Salt, craves—Nat mur

Scars easily—Silicea

Scars, keloid—Graphites

Sedentary—Nux vomica

Senses oversensitive—Coffea

Sensitive to drafts—Hepar sulph, Selenium

Sensitive to noise—Borax

Sensitive to others energy—Phosphorus, also Sepia

Sensitive to smell—Colchicum

Sensitive to temperature—Mercury sol

Sensitive to tobacco—Lobelia

Sex drive, low—Sepia

Sex drive, no sex drive—Graphites

Sexual abuse, history of—Staphysagria

Sexual excitement, poor function—Picric acid

Sexual problems—Sabal

Sharp pains worse with motion—Bryonia

Shellfish allergy—Urtica

Shingles—Mezereum, Ranunculus

Shock—Aconite, Arnica, Carbo veg, Gelsemium

Shoulder left—Ranunculus

Shoulder stiffness—Cimicifuga

Shy—Silicea

Sighing—Ignatia

Sinus infection—Kali bich

Sitting on a ball sensation, as if—Chimaphila

Skin—Calc sulph, Graphites, Mezereum, also Silicea

Skin burns—Calendula, Cantharis, also Causticum

Skin, brown spots—Kali sulph

Skin, calluses, hard, brittle—Antimonium crud

Skin, deep bloody skin cracks—Petroleum

Skin, fungal problems—Dulcamara

Skin, scabs with pus underneath, yellow oozing gluey—Mezereum

Skin, vitiligo (lack of skin pigmentation)—Kali sulph, also Arsenicum

Sleepless 1 to 3 A.M. with anxiety and fear—Kali ars

Sleeplessness due to busy mind-mind racing—Coffea

Slow pulse—Digitalis

Small intestine—Mag mur

Smell metallic—Mercury sol

Smell, rotten egg—Staphysagria, Sulphur

Smell, sensitive to—Colchicum

Sneezing—Sabadilla

Soft, organs or tissues—Calc fluor

Soreness—Hamamelis

Sour everything, attitude, smells etc.—Mag carb, also Calc carb

Sour food, craves—Sepia

Sour odors—Calc carb, also Mag carb

Spasms—Cuprum met, Hyoscyamus, Zincum

STD (sexually transmitted disease) problems, treated with antibiotics —Clematis

Stiffness better from continued motion—Rhus tox

Stimulants—Nux vomica

Stinging—Apis, Cantharis, Urtica

Stings or bites—Ledum, also Apis

Stomach sinking sensation—Ipecac

Stools, involuntary Muriatic acid

Stupor—Opium

Sudden symptoms—Belladonna

Suffocation sensation—Spongia

Sugar craving—Argentum nit

Suicidal—Aurum met

Sunburn—Cantharis

Sunstroke—Glonoinum, also Belladonna

Surgical cuts—Staphysagria

Sweat cold—Veratrum

Swelling—Apis

Tailbone injuries—Hypericum perf

Talkative—Lachesis

Taste, metallic—Mercury sol

Tears bland—Allium

Teeth—Fluoric acid

Teeth enamel deficient—Calc fluor

Teeth enamel deficient—Calc fluor

Teeth, cavities in—Calc fluor

Teething—Chamomilla

Temperature sensitive—Mercury sol

Tendonitis—Ruta

Test funk—Picric acid

Testicles—Aurum met

Thin—Calc phos

Thoughts, wild—Lilium tig

Throat constricted—Lachesis

Throat sore—Phytolacca dec

Throat, lump in—Ignatia

Throbbing—Belladonna

Thyroid—Spongia

Tobacco addiction—Clematis

Tobacco aggravates—Spigelia

Tobacco, sensitive to—Lobelia, also Ignatia

Tongue cankers—Borax

Travel, likes—Carcinosin

Tremors—Gelsemium

Twitching—Agaricus

Urinary leakage—Causticum

Urinary retention—Chimaphila

Urinary tract infections—Cantharis, Equisetum, Mercury corrosive, Staphysagria

Urination nightly frequent—Chimaphila

Urine smells like violets—Terebinthina

Urine strong smelling—Benzoic acid

Vaginal discharges corrosive—Kreosotum

Varicose veins—Aesculus

Vertigo—Muriatic acid, Tabacum, also Cocculus

Victims of violence—Stramonium

Violence, victims of—Stramonium

Voice, weak—Stannum met

Vomiting—Iris versicolor, Lobelia

Wandering symptoms—Pulsatilla

Warts—Dulcamara, Thuja, also Antimonium crud

Water regulator—Nat sulph

Weak ankles—Calc carb

Weak voice—Stannum met

Weakness—Stannum met

Weepy—Pulsatilla

Whooping cough—Drosera

Worse anger—Chamomilla

Worse antibiotics—Nitric acid

Worse before storms—Rhus tox

Worse cold—Spongia, also Rhus tox

Worse cold air—Sabadilla

Worse cold damp—Antimonium crud, also Rhus tox

Worse cold wind—Aconite

Worse dairy—Mag carb

Worse downward motion—Borax

Worse drafts—Kali carb

Worse dry—Spongia

Worse exposure to cold air—Rumex

Worse from 2 to 4 A.M.—Kali carb

Worse from 4 to 8 P.M.—Lycopodium

Worse heat—Secale

Worse night—Cuprum met

Worse smells—Sabadilla

Worse touch—Lac caninum, Nitric acid, Ruta

Worse waking—Lachesis

Worse winter—Petroleum

Worse with motion (sharp pains)—Bryonia

Wounds—Calendula, Ledum

Yellow discharges—Nat phos, Nat sulph

Yellow green discharges—Mercury sol, Kali bich, Thuja

Quick Reference Guide #3
Common Health Issues and Their Remedies

Each homeopathic remedy, in the Materia Medica Chapter 3, has a list of common health issues associated. This quick reference is a compilation of each common health issue and the remedies matching, according to symptom, in alphabetical order. Other remedies have been added that may also be helpful.

Abscesses—Calc sulph, Hepar sulph, Pyrogenium

Aching—Arnica, Hamamelis, Lactic acid

Acidity—Nat phos

Acne—Bovista, Calc sulph, Capsicum, Kali brom

Addiction, opiate—Ipecac, also Nux vomica

Addison's disease(adrenals)—Sepia, also Gelsemium

Alcoholism—Agaricus, Arsenicum, Aurum met, Chimaphila, Capsicum, Hyoscyamus, Lachesis (in females), Muriatic acid, Ranunculus, Sulphuric acid, Zincum, also Nux vomica (in males)

Allergic reactions (especially to shellfish)—Urtica

Allergies (hay fever)—Allium, Apis, Arsenicum, Arsenicum iod, Euphrasia, Kali ars, Kali mur, Nat mur, Sabadilla

Allergies, food—Merc sol

ALS (amyotrophic lateral sclerosis)—Alumina

Amenorrhea (lack of menstruation)—Ignatia

Anal deep skin cracks—Ledum, Nitric acid

Anemia—Calc ars, China/cinchona, Ferrum met, Pulsatilla, Rumex

Aneurysm—Lycopodium

Anger, suppressed—Staphysagria

Angina (heart pain)—Digitalis, Glonoinum, Mag phos, Spigelia

Ankles weak—Calc carb

Antibiotics (after)—Nitric acid

Anticipation—Argentum nit

Anxiety—Gelsemium, Kali ars, Spigelia

Appendicitis—Bryonia, also Belladonna

Arteriosclerosis—Aurum met

Arthritis—Aesculus, Bellis, Benzoic acid, Bryonia, Calc carb, Cimicifuga, Colchicum, Dulcamara, Ferrum met, Kali bich, Phytolacca, Rhus tox, Ruta grav, Sanguinaria, Urtica

Asphyxia—Antimonium tart, Carbo veg

Asthma—Arsenicum, Arsenicum iod, Carbo veg, Drosera, Kali ars, Kali carb, Lobelia, Nat sulph

Astigmatism—Lilium tig

Autism—Nat mur

Baby fat—Calc carb, Sepia

Back, discs herniated—Tellurium met, also Rhus tox

Back, herniated discs—Tellurium met, also Rhus tox

Backache—Aesculus, Kali carb, Ruta grav, also Rhus tox, Bryonia

Bad news—Gelsemium

Basedow's disease—Glonoinum

Bed sores—Lachesis, Muriatic acid, Pyrogenium, also Calendula

Bedwetting—Benzoic acid, Equisetum, Sabal, also Sepia

Bee stings—Apis

Belching—Antimonium crud, Carbo veg, Lycopodium, Mag carb

Bell's Palsy—Causticum, also Belladonna

Bipolar—Lachesis (in women)

Bites—Hypericum, Ledum, Pyrogenium, also Apis

Black eyes—Arnica, Ledum

Bladder—Berberis vulg, Cantharis, Merc corr, Terebinthina

Blindness, night—Helleborus

Bloating—Lycopodium

Blood disorders—Sanguinaria

Blood loss—China/cinchona

Blood poisoning—Crotalus horr, Hypericum, Kreosotum, Pyrogenium, also Lachesis

Blood pressure high—Aurum met, Benzoic acid, Lachesis, Nat mur

Blood problems—Ferrum met, also Phosphorus

Blows—Arnica

Boils—Arnica, Belladonna, Bellis, Lachesis, Picric acid, Hepar sulph, Phytolacca. See also abscesses.

Bone bruises—Ruta grav

Bone fractures—Symphytum

Bone problems—Calc carb, Calc phos, Fluoric acid

Bone spurs—Calc fluor, Calc phos

BPH (enlarged prostate)—Sabal. See also Prostate problems.

Brain bleeding—Sulphuric acid

Brain fog—Picric acid, Zincum

Brain injuries—Helleborus, also Nat sulph. See also Head injury.

Breast cancer—Conium, Carcinosin

Breast problems—Lactic acid, Phytolacca, also Conium

Breastfeeding—Phytolacca

Breasts painful—Lac caninum, also Phytolacca. See also mastitis.

Breathing difficult—Digitalis

Bronchitis—Antimonium tart, Drosera, Kali carb, Phosphorus, Rumex, Stannum met

Bruises—Bellis, Hamamelis, Ledum, Sulphuric acid, also Arnica

Bubonic plague—Crotalus horr. See also plague.

Burning pains—Arsenicum, Capsicum, Merc corr, also Phosphorus

Burns—Calendula, Cantharis, Causticum, Hamamelis, Kali bich, Sulphuric acid, Urtica

Calcification (hardening)—Calc fluor

Cancer, lung—Arsenicum iod

Cancer, prostate—Conium

Cancers, female—Sepia

Canker sores—Borax, Merc sol, Phosphoric acid

Carbon monoxide poisoning—Bovista, Carboneum sulph, Carbo veg

Carpal tunnel—Ruta grav

Cervical problems—Conium, also Thuja

Chicken pox—Pulsatilla, also Rhus tox

Chilliness—Sabadilla

Chills—Aconite

Cholera—Carbo veg, Cuprum met, Kreosotum, Veratrum

Chronic fatigue—Carcinosin, Cocculus, Gelsemium, Phosphoric acid, also Arsenicum

Cirrhosis of the liver—China/cinchona, Crotalus horr, Mag mur, also Phosphorus

Coffee abuse—Chamomilla

Colds—Allium, Dulcamara

Colds/flu—Aconite, Ferr phos, also Kali mur

Colic—Bovista, Chamomilla, Coffea, Colocynthis, Ignatia, Mag carb, Staphysagria

Colitis—Lycopodium, Staphysagria

Collapse—Carbo veg, Veratrum

Coma—Helleborus, Opium, Veratrum

Concussion—Arnica, Cicuta, Helleborus, Nat sulph

Confusion—Arnica

Constipation—Alumina, Crocus, Ferrum met, Mag mur, Sepia

Convulsions—Cicuta, Cuprum met, Ignatia, Zincum

Cough—Drosera, Ipecac, Kali carb, Rumex, Tellurium met

Cramps—Cuprum met, Ipecac, Mag phos

Croup—Aconite, Calc fluor, Spongia

Cuts—Calendula

Cyanosis (blueness)—Digitalis

Cysts—Bellis, Thuja, also Silicea

Dairy allergies—Mag carb, Mag mur

Dandruff—Kali sulph

Debility—Picric acid

Dehydration—Veratrum, also China/cinchona

Delirium—Belladonna Hyoscyamus

Delirium tremens—Nux vomica, Opium, Ranunculus

Delusions— Belladonna, Lac caninum, also Veratrum

Depression—Argentum nit, Ignatia, Kali phos, Lilium tig, Nat mur, Nat sulph

Diabetes—Calc carb, Carcinosin, Lactic acid, Lycopodium, Phosphoric acid, Phosphorus

Diarrhea—Bovista, Colchicum, Mag carb, Mag mur, Merc corr, Nat phos, Nitric acid, Phosphoric acid, Podophyllum

Difficult breathing—Digitalis

Digestive (GI) problems—Graphites

Digestive ulcers—Calendula, Fluoric acid, Kreosotum, Lachesis, Merc corr, Muriatic acid, Nat phos, Nitric acid, Sulphur

Digestive ulcers—Sulphur

Diphtheria—Lac caninum

Disappointment—Ignatia

Discharges offensive—Pyrogenium

Diuretic abuse—Equisetum

Drug addiction—Nux vomica, Muriatic acid

Drug overdose—Gelsemium

Dysentery—China/cinchona, Ipecac, Merc corr

Dyslexia—Lycopodium

Ear drums infected -Calendula

Ear problems—Pulsatilla, Kali mur

Earaches—Belladonna, Chamomilla, Pulsatilla

Ears, ringing (tinnitus)—China/cinchona, Cicuta

Eczema—Berberis vulg, Graphites, Kali ars, Kali sulph, Mezereum, Petroleum, Sulphur, Tellurium met

Edema (swelling)—Crotalus horr, Fluoric acid

Emaciation—Alumina, Arsenicum iod, China/cinchona, Nitric acid

Emphysema—Antimonium tart

Epididymitis (male genital inflammation), Sabal, Aurum met

Epilepsy—Calc ars, Calc carb, Cuprum met, Nat sulph, Zincum

Eustachian tubes—Ferr phos, Kali mur

Excitement—Coffea

Exhaustion, physical—Spongia, also Phosphoric acid

Eye injuries—Symphytum

Eye pains—Spigelia

Eye problems—Clematis, Pulsatilla, Spigelia

Eye strain—Ruta grav

Eyelid problems—Staphysagria

Eyelid swelling—Kali carb, Apis

Eyes weak from computer work—Euphrasia

Eyes, bleeding—Sulphuric acid

Eyes, cataracts—Apis, Calc fluor

Eyes, central vision— Carboneum sulph

Eyes, conjunctivitis—Euphrasia, Pulsatilla

Eyes, detached retina—Apis, also Phosphorus

Eyes, iritis—Merc corr

Eyes, double vision—Gelsemium

Eyes, photophobia—Nat sulph, Nux vomica

Eyes, strabismus (cross-eyed)—Cicuta

Facial hair in women—Sabal, also Sepia, Lycopodium

Facial nerve pains (neuralgia)—Mag phos

Facial paralysis—Causticum

Fainting—Tabacum, Veratrum

Fatigue—Kali phos

Fears—Aconite, Argentum nit, Opium

Fevers—Aconite, Ferr phos, Kali sulph, Muriatic acid, Pyrogenium, also Kali mur, Belladonna

Fissures (deep skin cracks)—Graphites

Fluoride poisoning—Fluoric acid

Food allergies—Merc sol

Food poisoning—Arsenicum, China/cinchona, Ipecac, also Nux vomica

Fright—Aconite, Gelsemium

Frostbite—Agaricus

Gallbladder—Bryonia, Pulsatilla, Sanguinaria

Gallstones—Berberis vulg

Ganglion cyst—Calc fluor, Ruta grav

Gangrene—Kreosotum, Secale, Sulphuric acid

Gas—Carcinosin, Carbo veg, Chamomilla, Colchicum, Lycopodium, Nat phos, Rumex, Sulphur, also Spongia

GI (digestive) problems—Graphites

Glandular swelling—Aesculus, Dulcamara, Phytolacca

Goiter—Fluoric acid, Spongia

Gonorrhea—Clematis, Merc corr

Gout—Antimonium crud, Benzoic acid, Colchicum, Urtica

Grief—Ignatia, Phosphoric acid, also Nat mur

Growing pains—Calc phos

Growths, non-cancerous—Thuja

Gunshot wounds—Symphytum

Hair loss—Selenium

Hallucinations—Belladonna, also Veratrum

Hangover—Nux vomica, Ranunculus

Hay fever (allergies)—Allium, Apis, Arsenicum, Arsenicum iod, Euphrasia, Kali ars, Kali mur, Nat mur, Sabadilla

Head injury—Arnica, Cicuta, Nat sulph, Veratrum, Zincum. See also brain injury.

Headaches—Iris versicolor, Kali bich, Picric acid, Sanguinaria, Zincum, also Ignatia

Heart attack—Aconite, also Lachesis

Heart disorders—Calc ars, Digitalis, Lachesis, Lilium tig, Spigelia

Heart failure—Spongia

Heart pain (angina)—Digitalis, Glonoinum, Mag phos, Spigelia

Heart palpitations—Aconite, Calc ars, Glonoinum Graphites Ignatia Mag mur, Pyrogenium, Spigelia

Heart, mitral valve—Digitalis

Heartburn—Carbo veg, Lobelia, Mag carb, Nat phos, Nux vomica, Sulphuric acid

Hemophilia (bleed easily)—Phosphorus, also Crotalus horr

Hemorrhage (excess bleeding)—Bovista, Cantharis, Carbo veg, Crocus, Crotalus horr, Ferrum met, Ferr phos, Hamamelis, Ipecac, Nitric acid, Secale, Terebinthina

Hemorrhoids—Aesculus, Hamamelis, Kali mur, Lycopodium, Muriatic acid, Nitric acid, Nux vomica

Hepatitis—Arsenicum Lycopodium Mag mur Nat sulph

Herpes—Borax, Dulcamara, Nat mur, Petroleum

High blood pressure—Aurum met, Benzoic acid, Lachesis, Nat mur

Hip joints—Aesculus

Hirsutism (excess facial hair in women), Sabal, also Sepia, Lycopodium

Hives—Apis, Nat phos, Urtica

Hoarseness—Causticum Kreosotum Stannum met

Homesickness—Capsicum, Phosphoric acid, also Ignatia

Hormonal disorders—Sepia, also Pulsatilla

Hot flashes—Cimicifuga, Digitalis, Sulphuric acid, also Sepia

Humiliation—Staphysagria

Hyperactive children—Arsenicum iod

Hypoglycemia—Lycopodium

Hysteria—Hyoscyamus, Ignatia

Impotence—Carboneum sulph, Nat mur, Selenium

Incontinence—Equisetum, Sabal, also Causticum

Incoordination—Argentum nit

Indigestion (pancreas)—Spongia

Infections—Belladonna, Clematis, Pyrogenium

Infertility—Nat mur, Sepia

Influenza—Gelsemium, also Aconite, Arsenicum. *See also* colds/flu

Injuries—Bellis, Bryonia, Calendula, Conium, Hypericum, Rhus tox, Tellurium met, also Arnica

Insanity—Hyoscyamus

Insomnia—Coffea, Kali phos, Mag carb

Intestinal cramps—Colocynthis

Itching—Mezereum

Jaundice—China/cinchona, Crotalus horr, Nat phos, Phosphorus

Joint pains—Bryonia, also Rhus tox

Joints dislocate—Ruta grav

Keloid scars—Carcinosin, also Graphites

Kidney inflammation (nephritis)—Apis, Berberis vulg, Terebinthina

Kidney pain—Berberis vulg, also Terebinthina

Kidney problems—Arsenicum , Calc ars, Equisetum, Merc corr, Picric acid, Terebinthina, also Berberis vulg

Kidney stones—Berberis vulg, Urtica

Labor disorders—Chamomilla

Labor pains—Coffea, also Cimicifuga, Pulsatilla

Lameness—Bellis, Ruta grav

Laryngitis—Causticum, Drosera

Leg with ankle swelling—Kali carb

Leukemia—Arsenicum

Lice—Sabadilla

Liver cirrosis—China/cinchona, Crotalus horr, Mag mur, also Nux vomica

Liver disorders or problems—Mag mur, Nat sulph, Nux vomica, Phosphorus

Locomotor Ataxia(can't walk properly), Secale

Lung cancer—Arsenicum iod

Lung weakness—Stannum met

Lupus—Kali bich

Lymphangitis—Bryonia, also Mercury sol

Lymphatics—Lactic acid, Pyrogenium

Macular degeneration—Bovista, also Calc ars, Carboneum sulph, Sepia

Malaria—Arsenicum, China/cinchona

Malnutrition—Calc carb, Mag carb

Mania—Belladonna, Hyoscyamus, Lachesis, Veratrum

Mastitis—Belladonna, Capsicum, Phytolacca

Masturbation, Phosphoric acid, Staphysagria

Measles—Euphrasia, Pulsatilla

Memory weakness—Picric acid

Meniere's disease—Benzoic acid

Meningitis—Apis, Cicuta, Cuprum met, Helleborus, Nat sulph, Opium, Veratrum, Zincum

Menopause—Cimicifuga, Lachesis, Sepia, also Graphites

Menstrual disorders—Chamomilla, Cimicifuga, also Sepia, Pulsatilla

Menstrual pain—Colocynthis, Mag mur

Menstruation, lack of—Pulsatilla

Mental disorders—Hyoscyamus

Mental fog—Kali phos, also Picricum acid

Migraine—Bryonia, Glonoinum, Iris versicolor, Kali bich, Lac caninum, Spigelia

Miscarriage—Ferrum met, Secale

Mononucleosis—Carcinosin, Dulcamara, Merc sol

Morning sickness—Colchicum, Ferrum met, Ipecac, Lactic acid, Nux vomica, Sepia, Tabacum

Motion sickness—Cocculus, Petroleum, Tabacum

Mucus—Allium, Kali bich, Kali mur, Kali sulph, Sabadilla

Multiple Sclerosis (MS)—Alumina, Argentum nit, Causticum, Colchicum, Conium, Merc sol, also Gelsemium

Mumps—Phytolacca, Pulsatilla, also Rhus tox

Muscle pains—Causticum

Muscle spasms—Zincum

Muscle weakness—Cocculus, Conium, Gelsemium

Nail fungus—Antimonium crud

Nail problems—Graphites

Nasal congestion—Dulcamara, Kali bich

Nausea—Colchicum, Ipecac, Iris versicolor, Lobelia, Nux vomica, Petroleum, Tabacum

Neck—Cimicifuga, Dulcamara

Nerve disorders—Mag mur, also Kali phos

Nerve weakness—Zincum

Nervous breakdown—Kali phos, also Ignatia

Nervous exhaustion—Picric acid

Neuralgia—Hypericum, Mezereum, Ranunculus

Neuritis—Urtica

Night blindness—Helleborus

Nightmares—Aconite, Stramonium

Nosebleeds—Crocus, Phosphorus, Secale, Stramonium

Nursing mothers—Cocculus

Nymphomania (hyper sexuality)—Hyoscyamus

Obesity—Calc ars, Graphites, also Calc carb

Obsessive compulsive—Carcinosin

Opiate addiction—Ipecac, also Nux vomica

Osteoporosis—Calc carb, Calc phos

Ovarian cysts—Colocynthis

Ovary problems—Lilium tig, also Lachesis

Pain, severe—Chamomilla

Pancreas—Calc ars, Phosphorus, also Spongia, Iris versicolor

Pancreatitis—Iris versicolor, also Spongia

Panic attacks—Aconite, Argentum nit, Kali ars

Paralysis—Causticum, Crotalus horr, Gelsemium, Mag phos, Opium, Zincum

Parasites—Calc carb, China/cinchona, Ignatia, Podophyllum, Sabadilla

Parkinson's with tremors—Merc sol

Peptic ulcers—Nat phos

Phantom limb pain—Symphytum, also Mag phos

Phlebitis (vein inflammation)—Hamamelis

Pinworms—Sabadilla

Plague—Crotalus horr

Pleurisy—Bryonia, Kali carb

Pneumonia—Antimonium tart, Arsenicum, Arsenicum iod, Bryonia, Kali carb, Phosphorus, Stramonium, Sulphur

Poison ivy—Ledum, also Rhus tox

Polyps—Calc carb, Carcinosin, Sanguinaria, Thuja, also Silicea

Post nasal drip—Kali bich

Post traumatic stress disorder (PTSD)—Opium, Stramonium, also Staphysagria

Proctitis, Nitric acid

Prostate cancer—Conium

Prostate problems—Chimaphila, Digitalis, Sabal, Selenium, also Conium

Psoriasis—Borax, Kali ars, Kali brom, Kali sulph, Graphites, Petroleum

Puncture wounds—Calendula, Ledum

Pus—Calc sulph, Hepar sulph, Silicea, also Pyrogenium

Putrid odor—Kreosotum

Rabies—Belladonna

Rape—Staphysagria

Rashes—Antimonium crud, Apis, Bovista, Dulcamara, Rhus tox, Urtica

Raynaud's disease (cold hands)—Secale

Religious delusions, as if evil or a servant of God— Kali brom, also Veratrum

Retina detached—Apis, also Phosphorus

Rib pain—Mag phos, Ranunculus

Rickets—Calc carb, Calc fluor, Phosphorus

Ringworm—Nitric acid, Tellurium met

Sacroiliac pain—Aesculus, Tellurium met, also Hypericum

Scars—Graphites, Silicea

Schizophrenia—Lachesis, also Veratrum

Sciatica—Colocynthis, Lycopodium, Mag phos, also Rhus tox, Hypericum

Scoliosis—Calc fluor, Calc phos, Silicea

Screaming—Chamomilla

Seasickness—Borax, Petroleum

Senility—Hyoscyamus

Sexual debility—Sabal

Sexual excess, Staphysagria

Shingles—Mezereum, Ranunculus

Shock—Carbo veg, Opium, Veratrum

Shoulders—Cimicifuga

Sighing—Ignatia

Sinusitis—Kali bich, Kali mur, Kali sulph, Sanguinaria

Skin calluses—Antimonium crud

Skin cracks—Petroleum

Skin eruptions—Mezereum

Skin hardening—Graphites

Skin problems—Graphites, Hepar sulph, Mezereum, Petroleum, Silicea. See also eczema and psoriasis.

Sleep deprivation—Cocculus

Sleeplessness—Coffea

Smell loss—Pulsatilla, also Nat mur, Mag mur

Sneezing—Allium, Sabadilla

Sore throat—Dulcamara, also Phytolacca

Spasms—Cuprum met, also Mag phos

Sperm, low count—Selenium

Spinal injuries—Hypericum, Nitric acid, also Rhus tox

Spinal irritation—Tellurium met

Spleen—China/cinchona

Splinter removal—Silicea

Sprains—Arnica, Ruta grav

Stage fright—Lycopodium, also Argentum nit

Stomach disorders—Nux vomica

Stomach ulcers—Muriatic acid

Strains—Arnica

Stroke—Arnica, Causticum, Crotalus horr, Glonoinum, Kali brom, Opium

Stuttering—Bovista, Causticum

Styes—Staphysagria

Suicidal—Aurum met, Nat sulph

Sunburn-Cantharis, also Causticum

Sunstroke—Glonoinum, Nat mur, Veratrum

Surgery—Calendula, Staphysagria

Sweat offensive—Tellurium met

Swelling—Bellis, also Crotalus horr, Fluoric acid

Swelling (edema)—Crotalus horr, Fluoric acid

Syphilis—Nitric acid

Tailbone injuries—Hypericum

Tears, excessive—Euphrasia

Teeth cavities—Calc fluor, also Calc phos

Teeth decay—Kreosotum

Teeth enamel, deficient—Calc fluor

Teeth problems—Fluoric acid

Teething—Calc carb, Chamomilla, Podophyllum

Tendon constriction—Causticum

Tendonitis—Bellis, Ruta grav

Testicle, right—Clematis

Testicles enlarged—Mezereum

Tetanus—Hypericum

Thrive, failure to—Mag carb

Throat disorders—Rumex

Throat sore—Dulcamara, also Phytolacca

Thrush—Borax

Thyroid disorders—Spongia

Tics—Agaricus

Tinnitus (ringing in ears)—China/cinchona, Cicuta

Tissue hardening—Graphites

Tobacco habit—Calc phos, Lobelia

Tonsillitis—Belladonna, Ferr phos, Lac caninum, Phytolacca

Toothache—Carboneum sulph, Clematis, Coffea, Mag phos

Toxemia—Apis

Trauma—Arnica, Opium

Trembling—Argentum nit, Conium

Tremors—Gelsemium, Ignatia

Trigeminal neuralgia—Spigelia. See also Neuralgia.

Tuberculosis—Drosera, Nitric acid

Tumors—Bellis, Calc fluor

Twitching—Agaricus, Ignatia

Typhoid fever—Muriatic acid

Ulcers, digestive—Calendula, Fluoric acid, Kreosotum, Lachesis, Merc
corr, Muriatic acid, Nat phos, Nitric acid, Sulphur

Ulcers, digestive—Sulphur

Unconsciousness—Coffea, also Opium

Urethritis—Digitalis

Urinary problems—Berberis vulg Picric acid

Urinary tract infection (UTI)—Cantharis, Chimaphila, Merc corr,
Sabal, Staphysagria, Terebinthina

Urination, frequent—Chimaphila, Equisetum

Urine retention—Terebinthina

Uterine problems—Lilium tig

Uterine prolapse—Lilium tig, Podophyllum, Sepia

Vaccinations—Belladonna, Carcinosin, Ledum, Thuja, also Silicea

Vaginal discharge—Graphites Kreosotum Mag carb Pulsatilla Secale

Vaginitis—Nat mur, Nat phos Pulsatilla, Sepia

Varicose veins—Aesculus, Calc fluor, Fluoric acid, Hamamelis

Vein inflammation (phlebitis)—Hamamelis

Veins, varicose ulcers—Hamamelis

Venereal warts—Thuja

Vertigo—Cocculus, Gelsemium, Opium, Petroleum, Stannum met, Tabacum

Victims of violence—Stramonium

Vitality low—Carbo veg

Vitiligo—Kali sulph, also Arsenicum

Voice, weak—Stannum met

Vomiting—Cocculus, Colchicum, Ipecac, Iris versicolor, Lobelia, Tabacum, also Nux vomica

Warts—Antimonium crud, Causticum, Dulcamara, Nitric acid, Thuja

Weakness—Gelsemium, Phosphoric acid

Whooping cough—Cuprum met, Drosera, Ipecac, Spongia

Worms—Nat phos

Worry—Ignatia

Wounds—Calendula, Hypericum, Lachesis, Ledum, Pyrogenium

Writer's cramp—Drosera

Yellow fever—Crotalus horr

Quick Reference Guide #4
Causations and Their Remedies

Causations are the reasons for the breakdown of the immune system, bringing on weakness and symptoms. The recommended homeopathic remedy or remedies will help the body recover from these causations. From emotions to cold winds, matching the causations with the right remedy will bring about harmony. In the list that follows, some remedies have been added that I have found to be helpful.

Abandonment—Pulsatilla

Abortion—Sepia

Abusive family—Thuja

Alcohol—Bryonia, Crotalus, Gelsemium, Kali bich, Nux vomica, Nat phos, Opium, Terebinthina

Alcoholism—Agaricus, Calc fluor, Digitalis, Lachesis, Lobelia, Sulphur

Allergens—Apis

Allergic tendencies—Arsenicum iod

Allergies (hay fever)—Euphrasia, Thuja

Anger—Antimonium tart, Mag mur

Angina (heart pain)—Glonoinum

Antibiotics—Nitric acid

Anticipation—Argentum nit

Anxiety—Kali ars

Arthritis—Thuja, also Rhus tox

Bee stings—Apis, see also Stings.

Betrayal—Nat mur

Birth control medications—Sepia

Bites—Arnica, Ledum, Tabacum

Blood loss—Carbo veg, China/cinchona, Ferrum met, Ferrum phos, Ipecac

Bone problems—Calc phos

Bones, broken—Symphytum

Brain injury—Zinc, also Nat sulph, *see also* Head injury

Burns—Calendula, Cantharis, Causticum, Sulphuric acid, Urtica

Business loss—Colocynthis, Kali brom

Cancer, family history—Carcinosin

Carbon monoxide poisoning—Bovista, Carbo veg, Carboneum sulph, Opium

Caretaking—Colchicum, Nitric acid, Zinc, also Ignatia

Celibacy—Conium, Lilium

Cellars, damp—Terebinthina, also Rhus tox

Childbirth—Bellis, Lilium, Sepia

Cold air, exposure to—Mag phos, Rumex

Cold damp—Allium cepa, Borax, Dulcamara, Nat sulph

Cold stormy weather—Rhus tox

Cold wind—Aconite, Bryonia, Hepar sulph

Computer work—Euphrasia

Concussion—Helleborus, also Nat sulph

Contradiction—Aurum met

Damp weather, exposure to—Phytolacca, also Rhus tox

Debilitating events—Selenium

Dehydration—China/cinchona

Dental work—Hypericum

Depletion from alcohol or other drug addictions—Muriatic acid

Diphtheria—Lac caninum

Disappointed honor—Veratrum

Disappointed love—Antimonium crud, Aurum met, Calc phos, Ignatia, Nat mur, Veratrum

Disappointment—Alumina

Discharges, suppression of—Secale

Diseases, chronic—Pyrogenium

Diuretic chronic use or abuse—Equisetum

Drafts—Belladonna, also Hepar sulph

Drug abuse—Gelsemium, Nux vomica, Phosphoric acid, Selenium, Veratrum

Drug addictions—Lobelia

Dusty wind—Euphrasia

Earaches—Chamomilla, also Kali Mur

Eczema, suppressed—Mezereum

Electricity—Stramonium, also Phosphorus

Electrocution—Phosphorus

Electroshock therapy—Phosphorus

Emotional losses—Ignatia, also Nat mur

Emotional trauma—Cimicifuga, Colchicum, Mag carb, Picric acid, Zinc, also Nat mur

Emotions—Apis, Coffea, Glonoinum, Lachesis, Mag phos, Phytolacca, Stannum, also Ignatia

Emotions, suppressed—Cuprum

Fats, eating—Pulsatilla

Fats, excessive—Ipecac

Fibroid problems—Spongia

Financial loss—Arsenicum, Aurum met

Fluid loss—Phosphoric acid, also China/cinchona

Fluoride deficiency—Fluoric acid

Food poisoning—Arsenicum, China/cinchona

Food tainted—Carbo veg

Foreign objects in the body—Silicea

Fright—Aconite, Crotalus, Gelsemium, Hyoscyamus, Lycopodium, Merc sol, Opium

Frostbite—Agaricus

Frustration—Colocynthis, Ipecac, Kali phos, Mag mur

Gas—Chamomilla

Gonorrhea—Merc sol, Thuja

Gonorrhea, suppressed from antibiotics—Merc corr

Grief—Graphites, Hyoscyamus, Nat mur, Phytolacca, also Ignatia

Growing too rapidly—Phosphoric acid

Hair cutting—Belladonna

Hamstrings—Ruta

Hay fever(allergies)—Euphrasia, Thuja

Head injury—Cicuta, Helleborus, Nat mur, Nat sulph, Spigelia

Head sweat—Belladonna

Hemorrhages—Secale

Hemorrhoids—Aesculus

Homesickness—Capsicum, Clematis

Hormonal imbalances (estrogen)—Sepia

Hormones, anything that changes—Sepia

Hot weather, taking cold in—Bryonia

Humiliation—Staphysagria

Infection with pus—Pyrogenium

Injuries—Arnica, Bellis, Bryonia, Calendula, Crocus, Ferrum phos, Hepar sulph, Ipecac, Kali mur, Kali phos, Kali sulph, Ledum, Mag carb, Phytolacca, Ruta, Silicea, Sulphuric acid, Symphytum, Tellurium, Terebinthina, Veratrum, also Rhus tox

Insect bites—Tabacum

Jealousy—Hyoscyamus

Joint injury—Rhus tox

Kidney problems—Benzoic acid, also Berberis vulg

Labor disorders—Chamomilla

Laxative abuse—Nux vomica

Liver problems—Podophyllum, also Nux vomica

Loss, financial—Arsenicum, Aurum met

Love loss—Helleborus, Hyoscyamus

Love, disappointed—Antimonium crud, Aurum met, Calc phos, Ignatia, Nat mur, Veratrum

Lung weakness—Rumex

Masturbation—Gelsemium, Lachesis, Stannum

Menopause—Aesculus, Lachesis, Lilium, also Graphites, Calc carb

Menstrual disorders—Chamomilla, also Sepia

Mental overwork—Kali phos, Picric acid, Sabadilla

Middle child doesn't feel appreciated—Calc sulph

Miscarriage—Pyrogenium, Secale

Motion sickness—Cocculus, Petroleum

Muscle overuse—Mag phos, also Arnica

Near-death experience—Opium

Nerve injuries—Hypericum

Nursing mothers—Cocculus

Nymphomania (hypersexuality)—Sabadilla

Obesity in menopausal women—Calc ars

Over-excitement—Agaricus

Over-exertion—Alumina

Over-heating in sun—Antimonium crud, also Belladonna

Over-lifting—Calc carb, Graphites

Over-study—Phosphoric acid, Selenium

Over-work—Bellis, Calc carb

Pain, severe—Chamomilla

Parasites—Sabadilla, Spigelia

Petroleum toxicity—Petroleum

Pleasure emotions—Coffea

Pneumonia, never well since—Kali carb, Sulphur

Poor diet—Nat phos

Poor nutrition—Calc carb, Mag carb

Poverty—Arsenicum

Pregnancy—Sepia

Prescription medications—Nux vomica

Puncture wounds—Ledum

Punishment—Staphysagria

Purgatives (never well since taking)—Sulphur

Pus with infection—Pyrogenium

Rape—Opium, Staphysagria

Rashes—Urtica

Reading, excess—Euphrasia

Rib injury—Ranunculus

Rich foods—Carbo veg

Rich living—Digitalis

Scalds—Causticum

Screaming—Chamomilla

Security, lack of—Calc sulph

Sexual abuse—Carcinosin, Digitalis, Sepia, also Staphysagria

Sexual excess—Argentum nit, Calc phos, Colocynthis, Conium, Kali brom, Lilium, Mag mur, Phosphoric acid, Sabal, Selenium, also Sepia

Shame—Staphysagria

Shellfish—Urtica

Shock—Gelsemium

Shock, post-operative—Veratrum

Sibling rivalry—Calc sulph

Skin conditions, suppressed from steroid creams—Hepar sulph, Kali carb, Petroleum

Sleep loss—Cocculus, Lachesis, Nitric acid, Zinc

Smoking—Lactic acid, Lobelia

Spinal injury—Rhus tox, Thuja

Splinters—Arnica, Silicea

Stimulant abuse of coffee or opiates—Chamomilla

Stings—Arnica, Ledum, Urtica

Strains—Calc carb

Sugar—Argentum nit, Ipecac, Lycopodium

Sun exposure—Nat mur, Spigelia, Tabacum, also Belladonna, Glonoinum

Sun overheating—Antimonium crud, also Belladonna, Glonoinum

Sunstroke—Belladonna, Glonoinum

Surgery—Arnica, Graphites, Staphysagria, Sulphuric acid

Sweat—Merc sol

Sweat suppressed—Colchicum

Sweating, taking cold from—Sanguinaria

Sweets, ailments from—Lycopodium, *see also* Sugar.

Taking cold from sweating—Sanguinaria

Taking cold in hot weather—Bryonia

Teething—Borax, Chamomilla, Stannum

Temperature extremes—Kali sulph

Tendon overuse—Ruta

Tobacco—Nux vomica, Spigelia

Tooth extraction—Terebinthina

Tuberculosis, family history of—Drosera

Urinary tract infection—Cantharis, also Staphysagria

Vaccinations—Antimonium tart, Carcinosin, Crotalus, Kali mur, Mezereum, Silicea, Thuja

Veins, varicose—Aesculus

Violence exposure to—Stramonium

Voice overuse—Stannum

Weather, cold damp—Allium cepa, also Rhus tox

Weather, cold stormy—Rhus tox

Wet, getting—Bellis, Rhus tox, Stramonium

Whooping cough, after—Sanguinaria

Wind, cold—Aconite

Wind, dusty—Euphrasia

Wine, ailments from—Lycopodium

Worried—Causticum, Kali brom

Wounds—Conium

Quick Reference Guide #5
Remedies and Their Conditions

This Quick Reference Guide briefly notes each homeopathic remedy and the conditions for which they are applied, as described in full detail in Chapter 3, Materia Medica. Additional descriptions have been added to help with differentiation.

Aconite—anxiety, cough, depression, fever, nerve pain, teething, tooth-aches, urinary tract infections

Aesculus hipp—hemorrhoids, also hips, excessive bleeding

Agaricus—nose bleeds, tremors, vision issues

Allium—hay fever, vision issues

Alumina—constipation, also elderly, fatigue, emaciation, memory issues

Antimonium crud—blisters, warts, also plantar warts, corns, indigestion

Antimonium tart—bronchitis, coughs, pneumonia, also rattling coughs

Apis—arthritis, bites and stings, blisters, conjunctivitis, incontinence, macular degeneration, also anaphylactic shock

Argentum nit—anxiety, bedwetting, conjunctivitis, gas, incontinence, sore throat, urinary tract infections, also panic attacks

Arnica—abscess/boils, back pain, bites and stings, blisters, bruising, ex-haustion, gout, head injury, injuries, muscle cramps, varicose veins

Arsenicum album—anxiety, asthma, bedwetting, bites and stings, burns, canker sores, cold sores, conjunctivitis, depression, diarrhea, eczema, exhaustion, flu, hay fever, heartburn, hemorrhoid, inconti-nence, leg ulcers, mucus, nerve pain, palpitations, pneumonia, pso-riasis, sleep problems, teething

Arsenicum iod—hay fever, also athlete's foot, lung problems

Aurum met—addiction, depression, grief, obesity, also suicidal feeling

Belladonna—arthritis, bites and stings, burns, earache, fever (high), headaches, incontinence, menstrual issues, mucus, muscle cramps, nerve pain, PMS, sore throats, teething, toothaches, urinary tract infections

Bellis—bruising, injuries, also bone bruising and tendonitis

Benzoic acid—gout, also strong-smelling urine, kidneys

Berberis vulg—gallstones, also kidney stones, radiating pains

Borax—canker sores, teething, also motion sickness

Bovista—macular degeneration, also rashes, acne

Bryonia—arthritis, back pain, bronchitis, coughs, flu, gout, headaches, injuries, pneumonia, sciatica, toothaches

Calc ars—macular degeneration, also obesity, pancreas

Calc carb—back pain, eczema, gallstones, gums, heartburn, hot flashes, menopause, mononucleosis, muscle cramps, obesity, palpitations, PMS, sore throats, sweating, teething, warts

Calc fluor—also cataracts, poor teeth enamel

Calc phos—teething, toothaches, also cavities, growing pains

Calc sulph—abscesses/boils, also skin problems

Calendula—burns, diaper rash, menopause

Cantharis—blisters, burns, urinary tract infections

Capsicum—obesity, sleep problems, also homesickness

Carbo veg—bloating, colic in babies, gas, gums, heartburn, hemorrhoids, leg ulcers, mucus, pneumonia, varicose veins

Carboneum sulph—macular degeneration, vision issues (central vision)

Carcinosin—mononucleosis

Causticum—bedwetting, blisters, bloating, burns, hemorrhoids, incontinence, itching, tremors, urinary tract infections, warts

Chamomilla—colic, earache, teething, toothache

Chimaphila—also kidney, bladder, urinary tract infections, prostate

Cicuta—head injury, also convulsions, epilepsy

Cimicifuga—depression, hot flashes, menopause, menstrual issues

China/cinchona—addictions, bloating, exhaustion, gallstones, sweating, toothaches

Clematis—shingles, also male genitals

Cocculus—nausea and vomiting, travel sickness, also vertigo

Coffea—sleep problems, toothaches, also insomnia, racing mind

Colchicum—gout, nausea and vomiting

Colocynthis—colic in babies, gallstones, gas, menstrual issues, nerve pain, PMS, sciatica

Conium—heartburn, PMS, prostate, travel sickness, also vertigo, breast problems

Crocus—hemorrhages

Crotalus horr—nosebleeds, also hemorrhages

Cuprum met—asthma, coughs, muscle cramps, tremors, also epilepsy (night)

Digitalis—slow heart rate, heart problems

Drosera—bronchitis, coughing, also whooping cough, asthma

Dulcamara—warts (flat), also stiff neck, rashes

Equisetum—bedwetting, also kidneys

Euphrasia—vision issues

Ferrum met—obesity, PMS, also low iron

Ferrum phos—fever, nosebleeds, also low iron

Fluoric acid—varicose veins, also teeth problems

Gelsemium—anxiety, exhaustion, fever, flu, macular degeneration, mononucleosis, vision issues, also panic attacks, internal shaking

Glonoinum—headaches, also migraines

Graphites—diaper rash, eczema, hot flashes, hypoglycemia, menopause, obesity, PMS

Hamamelis—bruising, hemorrhoids, nosebleeds, varicose veins

Helleborus—head injury, also meningitis

Hepar sulph—abscesses/boils, acne, coughs, earaches, eczema, sleep problems, sweating

Hyoscyamus—also alcoholism, hysteria, hypersexual

Hypericum—back pain, bites and stings, head injury, injuries, nerve pain

Ignatia—depression, grief, headaches, menstrual issues, nerve pain, PMS, sore throat

Ipecac—asthma, cough, morning sickness, nausea and vomiting, PMS

Iris versicolor—headaches, shingles, also pancreas

Kali ars—anxiety, sleep problems, also panic attacks

Kali bich—burns, mucus(thick), obesity, sinus

Kali brom—acne, muscle cramps

Kali carb—arthritis, asthma, bloating, hypoglycemia, menstrual issues, obesity, sleep problems

Kali mur—fever (medium), also Eustachian tube blockage, respiratory

Kali phos—depression, exhaustion, gums

Kali sulph—earaches, fever (high)

Kreosotum—bedwetting, gums, mucus, also vaginitis

Lac caninum—PMS, also breast pain, uterine disorders

Lachesis—abscesses/boils, addictions, bites and stings, depression, gums, headaches, hemorrhoids, hot flashes, leg ulcers, macular degeneration, menopause, nosebleeds, PMS, sore throats

Lactic acid—morning sickness, also muscle pains

Ledum—bites and stings, bruising, also anal fissures, puncture wounds

Lilium tig—depression, also heart problems, female complaints

Lobelia—asthma, nausea and vomiting, pneumonia

Lycopodium—back pain, bedwetting, bloating, gallstones, gas, gout, headaches, heartburn, hypoglycemia, incontinence, leg ulcers, psoriasis, sinus, sore throat, sweating, varicose veins

Mag carb—also gas, bloating, heartburn

Mag mur—also small intestine, constipation or diarrhea, gas, liver problems

Mag phos—colic in babies, menstrual issues, muscle cramps, nerve pain, PMS, sciatica, also phantom limb pains

Mercury corr—cankers, diaper rash, gums, urinary tract infections

Mercury sol/vivus—abscesses/boils, cankers, diaper rash, earaches, gums, mononucleosis, morning sickness, mucus, pneumonia, shingles, sinus, sore throat, teething, toothaches

Mezereum—eczema, itching, shingles

Muriatic acid—diaper rash, also hemorrhoids, exhaustion

Nat mur—back pain, cold sores, constipation, depression, grief, gums, hay fever, incontinence, menopause, mucus, palpitations, PMS, psoriasis, shingles, sweating

Nat phos—also heartburn, peptic ulcers, parasites, hives

Nat sulph—asthma, depression, diarrhea, gallstones, gas, hay fever, head injury, injuries, vision issues, also convulsions

Nitric acid—gums, hemorrhoids, mucus, sore throats, vision issues, warts, also anal fissures

Nux vomica—acne, addictions, back pain, canker sores, colic in babies, constipation, coughs, gas, gout, heartburn, hemorrhoids, morning sickness, muscle cramps, nausea and vomiting, sleep problems, sweating, travel sickness, tremors, urinary tract infections, also alcoholism (males)

Opium—PTSD, constipation, paralysis, post stroke

Petroleum—eczema, itching, travel sickness

Phosphoric acid—exhaustion, grief, palpitations

Phosphorus—anxiety, bloating, bronchitis, bruising, burns, coughs, diarrhea, gas, gums, heartburn, hypoglycemia, macular degeneration, mucus, nosebleeds, palpitations, PMS, pneumonia, sweating, vision issues

Picric acid—exhaustion, also test fears, memory issues

Phytolacca—PMS, psoriasis, also sore throat, mastitis

Podophyllum—diarrhea, also teething, uterine or rectal prolapse

Pulsatilla—bedwetting, conjunctivitis, coughs, depression, earaches, grief, headaches, hot flashes, incontinence, menopause, menstrual issues, morning sickness, mucus, palpitations, PMS, prostate, sinus, urinary tract infections, varicose veins

Pyrogenium—burns, also infections, pus

Ranunculus—shingles, also rib injuries

Rhus tox—acne, arthritis, back pain, blisters, cold sores, conjunctivitis, eczema, flu, gout, injuries, itching, sciatica, shingles, sleep issues

Rumex—bronchitis, coughs

Ruta—bruising, injuries, also tendonitis, ganglion cysts, carpel tunnel

Sabadilla—hay fever, also sneezing

Sabal—prostate, also bedwetting, impotence, prostate disorders

Sanguinaria—headaches (right-sided), also shoulder (right) arthritis

Secale—nosebleeds, also hemorrhages, instability

Selenium—prostate, male sex problems

Sepia—acne, back pain, bedwetting, cold sores, constipation, depression, hot flashes, incontinence, macular degeneration, menopause, menstrual issues, morning sickness, mucus, obesity, sweating

Silica—abscesses/boils, acne, arthritis, cold sores, constipation, earaches, exhaustion, gums, headaches, hypoglycemia, mucus, PMS, sinus, sleep problems, sweating, teething

Spigelia—headaches (left), nerve pain, palpitations, also heart problems, neuralgia

Spongia—bronchitis, cough, also pancreatitis

Stannum met—bronchitis, also exhaustion

Staphysagria—grief, injuries, prostate, psoriasis, toothaches, urinary tract infections, also rape, child abuse, bulimia, self-mutilation.

Stramonium—also nightmares, victims of violence, violent

Sulphur—acne, back pain, canker sores, cold sores, conjunctivitis, diaper rash, diarrhea, eczema, hemorrhoids, hypoglycemia, itching, PMS

Sulphuric acid—bruising, canker sores, diaper rash, head injury, vision issues, also bleeding in eyes or brain

Symphytum—injuries (bone), also wounds, eye injuries, phantom limb pains

Tabacum—nausea and vomiting, travel sickness

Tellurium met—sciatica, also low back pain or injury

Terebinthina—urinary tract infections, also kidney problems

Thuja—acne, prostate, sinus, warts, also abnormal non-cancerous growths

Urtica—bites and stings, also hives, rashes

Veratrum—diarrhea, muscle cramps, also religious delusions

Zinc—muscle cramps, tremors, varicose veins, also convulsions

Index

Please consult the **Table of Contents**, pages ix-xii.

Page listings for the major health **Conditions** covered in this book are presented under Chapter 2; page listings for **Homeopathic remedies** are presented under Chapter 3.

Additionally, health Conditions are arranged alphabetically in Chapter 2; Homeopathic remedies are arranged alphabetically in Chapter 3; with names at the top of each page for the Conditions or Remedies covered there.

References

Nature's Materia Medica, 3rd Edition, 2006
Robin Murphy, N.D.
Lotus Health Institute

Homeopathic Clinical Repertory, 3rd Edition 2005
Robin Murphy, N.D.
Lotus Health Institute

Prisma, 2002
Franz Vermeulen
Emryss bu Publishers

Physical Examination and Observations in Homeopathy, 1992
Filip Degroote, M.D.
Homeoden Book Service

Desktop Guide to Keynotes and Confirmatory Symptoms, 1993
Roger Morrison, M.D.
Hahnemann Clinic Publishing

The Spirit of Homeopathy, 2nd Edition, 1994
Rajan Sankaran
Homeopathic Medical Publishers, Bombay

Resources

PRODUCTS:

To purchase homeopathic medicines (Boiron or Hylands), or to make an appointment for a homeopathic consultation (over the phone or in-person) with Dave Card, contact us at Dave's Health & Nutrition, 880 E 3900 S, Salt Lake City, Utah 84107, Phone: 801-268-3900, or see our website at *www.DavesHealth.com*.

Washington Homeopathic Products at *www.homeopathyworks.com* for a full line of homeopathic singles and supplies.

ABC Homeopathics at *www.abchomeopathy.com* for remedies and an online remedy finder.

BOOKS:

Learn more about Cell Salts through Dave's books:
Facial Diagnosis of Cell Salt Deficiencies (Kalindi Press, 2005)
and *12 Essential Minerals for Cellular Health* (Kalindi Press, 2007)

ONGOING EDUCATION:

www.DavesHealingNotes.com is your source for homeopathic solutions, helping various conditions and diseases.

For more education on using homeopathic medicines, offered by Dave Card, see the following seminars at *www.DavesHealth.com/daves-seminars*:

- Emotional Healing With Herbs and Homeopathy
- Facial Diagnosis
- The Power of Cell Salts
- Practical Homeopathy
- Seven Symbols of Healing

Contact Information

ABOUT THE AUTHOR

DAVID ROBERT CARD: Born in Alberta, Canada, and currently at home in Sandy, Utah, Dave Card continues to be active in his community and nationally through teaching and a highly respected homeopathy practice developed over thirty years. He holds a degree in psychology from the University of Utah, and certifications from numerous agencies including the National Institute of Nutritional Education, the Hahnemannian Institute of Homeopathy, and the School of Natural Healing. He is owner of Dave's Health and Nutrition, two stores, and actively creates online courses, and books on a wide variety of health-related topics. He has authored two bestselling books for Kalindi Press: *Facial Diagnosis of Cell Salt Deficiencies*, and *12 Essential Minerals*.

Contact Information: *Daveshealth.com* and *Daveshealingnotes.com*

ABOUT KALINDI PRESS

KALINDI PRESS, an affiliate of HOHM PRESS, proudly offers books in natural health and nutrition, as well as the acclaimed Family and World Health Series for children and parents, covering such themes as nutrition, dental health, reading and environmental education.

Contact Information: Kalindi Press, PO Box 4410, Chino Valley, Arizona, 86323; USA; 800-381-2700, or 928-636-3331; email: *publisher@ hohmpress.com*

Visit our website at: *www.kalindipress.com*